Natural Solutions for Diabetes

Srivastava Shikha

Copyright © 2024 by Srivastava Shikha

All rights reserved. No part of this book may be reproduced in any manner whatsoever without written permission except in the case of brief quotations embodied in critical articles and reviews.

First Printing, 2024

CONTENTS

Page No.

Abstract
List of Tables
List of Figures
List of Symbols and Abbreviations

CHAPTER 1: INTRODUCTION — 2-26

CHAPTER 2: AIM AND OBJECTIVE OF WORK — 28-31

CHAPTER 3: LITERATURE REVIEW — 33-72

CHAPTER 4: MATERIALS AND METHODS — 73-87

CHAPTER 5: RESULTS AND OBSERVATIONS — 89-205

CHAPTER 6: DISCUSSION — 207-208

CHAPTER 7: CONCLUSION AND DIRECTION FOR FUTURE USE — 210-212

LIST OF TABLES

Table No.	TITLE	PAGE No.
3.1	Summary of the history of diabetes	33
3.2	Oral hypoglycemic drugs act by different mechanism to control the condition of hyperglycemia	36
3.3	Phytochemicals with their reported mode of action in managing the diabetes	40
3.4	Phytoconstituents with their common prominent mode of action	43
3.5	Summary of antidiabetic plants whose study has already been conducted on STZ induced diabetic rats	44
3.6	List of Polyherbal Formulations with their composition and tested dose for antidiabetic activity	48
3.7	Phytochemical Review on Isolated Phytoconstituents from *Morus alba*	53
3.8	Pharmacological Activities of *Morus alba*	54
3.9	Phytochemical Review on Isolated Phytoconstituents from *Annona squamosa*	55
3.10	Pharmacological Activities of *Annona squamosa*	56
3.11	Phytochemical Review on Isolated Phytoconstituents from *Nelumbo nucifera*	57
3.12	Pharmacological Activities of *Nelumbo nucifera*	58
3.13	Phytochemical Review on Isolated Phytoconstituents from *Psidium guajava*	59
3.14	Pharmacological Activities of *Psidium guajava*	60
3.15	Phytochemical Review on Isolated Phytoconstituents from *Coccinia indica*	61
3.16	Pharmacological activities of *Coccinia indica*	61
3.17	Phytochemical Review on Isolated Phytoconstituents from *Gymnema sylvestre*	62
3.18	Pharmacological activities of *Gymnema sylvestre*	63

3.19	Phytochemical Review on Isolated Phytoconstituents from *Pterocarpus marsupium*	64
3.20	Pharmacological activities of *Pterocarpus marsupium*	64
3.21	Phytochemical Review on Isolated Phytoconstituents from *Syzium cumini*	65
3.22	Pharmacological activities of *Syzium cumini*	66
3.23	Phytochemical Review on Isolated Phytoconstituents from *Momordica charantia*	68
3.24	Pharmacological activities of *Momordica charantia*	68
3.25	Phytochemical Review on Isolated Phytoconstituents from *Piper longum*	70
3.26	Pharmacological activities of *Piper longum*	70
4.1	Preliminary Phytochemical screening of Plants by different chemical test	75
4.2	Preliminary Phytochemical screening of Plants by different chemical test	77
4.3	Design of Polyherbal formulations on the basis of targeted sites of action	78
4.4	Design of Polyherbal formulations on the basis of targeted sites of action (with equal doses of each extract)	79
5.1	Results of Physico-chemical evaluation of the plant material	89
5.2	Results of Physicochemical evaluation of the plant material	90
5.3	Percentage yield of hydro-alcoholic plant extracts	90
5.4	Results of Preliminary Phytochemical screening of Plants	91
5.5	Results of Preliminary Phytochemical screening of Plants	91
5.6	Results of Toxicity study of formulation A	92
5.7	Results of Toxicity study of Formulation B	92
5.8	Results of Toxicity study of Formulation C	93
5.9	Results of Toxicity study of Formulation D	93
5.10	Results of Toxicity study of Formulation E	94
5.11	Results of Toxicity study of Formulation F	94
5.12	Results of Oral glucose tolerance test	95

5.13	Oral glucose tolerance test (Blood glucose level expressed in Mean± S.E)	97
5.14	Effect of Polyherbal formulations on change in Blood glucose level and body weight from 0 day to 15th days (n=5)	102
5.15	Effect of Polyherbal formulations on change in Fasting Blood glucose level in albino wistar rats 0 to 15 days (Mean ± S.D) n=5	105
5.16	Total decrease in Percentage (%) of Average Blood glucose level from 0 day to 15th day for all six Poly herbal formulations	106
5.17	Effect of Polyherbal formulation A (FA) on change in biochemical parameters of blood plasma in albino wistar rats from 0 day to 15th day	109
5.18	Effect of Polyherbal formulation B (FB) on change in biochemical parameters of blood plasma in albino wistar rats from 0 day to 15th day	111
5.19	Effect of Polyherbal formulation C (FC) on change in biochemical parameters of blood plasma in albino wistar rats from 0 day to 15th day	113
5.20	Effect of Polyherbal formulation D (FD) on Change in biochemical parameters of blood plasma in albino wistar rats from 0 day to 15th day	115
5.21	Effect of Polyherbal formulation E (FE) on Change in biochemical parameters of blood plasma in albino wistar rats from 0 day to 15th day	117
5.22	Effect of Polyherbal formulation F (FF) on Change in biochemical parameters of blood plasma in albino wistar rats from 0 day to 15th day n=5	119
5.23	Effect of Formulations on Biochemical Parameters of blood plasma. Values are showed in mean ± SE from 5 animals in each group	121
5.24	Effect of Formulations on Biochemical Parameters of blood. Values are mean ± SE from 5 animals in each group	123
5.25	Average Percentage decreases in Biochemical parameters of blood serum of diabetic rats from 0 to 15th days for all the six Formulations	125
5.26	Analysis of other Biochemical Parameters	127
5.27	Results of Heavy metal content determination in Polyherbal formulations by Atomic absorption Spectroscopy.	203
5.28	Results of Microbial Load in Polyherbal Formulation (FA-FF)	204

LIST OF FIGURES

Figure No.	TITLE	PAGE No.
1.1	Countries with higher number of Diabetes subjects in year 2015	3
1.2	Countries with higher number of Diabetes subjects in year 2030	4
1.3	Prevalence of Diabetes in different parts of India	4
1.4	Type 1 Diabetes mellitus	8
1.5	Type 2 Diabetes mellitus	10
1.6	Gestational diabetes	11
1.7	Symptoms of Diabetes	12
1.8	Panchmahabhoot (5 elements)	13
3.1	Antidiabetic activity distributed in plants parts	47
4.1	Extraction by using Soxhlet's apparatus	75
5.1	Average decrease in percentage in Blood Glucose Level from 0 to 15th day	108
5.2	Average % decrease in biochemical parameters from 0 to 15th day	126
5.3	Average % decrease in biochemical parameters from 0 to 15th day	126
5.4	Chromatogram of Standard Quercetin, Rutin and Stigma sterol at 254 nm	132
5.5	Chromatogram of Standard Gallic acid, Ellagic acid, Catechin and Epicatechin at 254 nm	133
5.6	Chromatogram of Standard Piperine, Polyherbal FA (f1), FB (f2) and FC (f3) at 254 nm	134
5.7	Chromatogram of Polyherbal FD (f4), FE (f5) and FF (f6) at 254 nm	135
5.8	Peak list of standard compound at 254 nm	137
5.9	Peak list of Polyherbal Formulations at 254 nm	139
5.10	Chromatogram of Quercetin at 254 nm	140
5.11	Chromatogram of Rutin at 254 nm	141
5.12	Chromatogram of Stigma sterol at 254 nm	142
5.13	Chromatogram of Gallic acid at 254 nm	143

5.14	Chromatogram of Ellagic acid at 254 nm	144
5.15	Chromatogram of Catechin at 254 nm	145
5.16	Chromatogram of Epicatechin at 254 nm	146
5.17	Chromatogram of Piperine at 254 nm	147
5.18	Chromatogram of Polyherbal formulation FA (f1) at 254 nm	148
5.19	Chromatogram of Polyherbal formulation FB (f2) at 254 nm	149
5.20	Chromatogram of Polyherbal formulation FC (f3) at 254 nm	150
5.21	Chromatogram of Polyherbal formulation FD (f4) at 254 nm	151
5.22	Chromatogram of Polyherbal formulation FE (f5) at 254 nm	152
5.23	Chromatogram of Polyherbal formulation FF (f6) at 254 nm	153
5.24	Chromatogram of Standard Quercetin, Rutin and Stigma sterol at 366 nm	156
5.25	Chromatogram of Gallic acid, Ellagic acid, Catechin and Epicatechin at 366 nm	157
5.26	Chromatogram of Piperine, Polyherbal FA (f1), FB (f2) and FC (f3) at 366 nm	158
5.27	Chromatogram of Polyherbal FD (f4), FE (f5) and FF (f6) at 366 nm	159
5.28	Peak list of Standards and Polyherbal Formulations at 366 nm	162
5.29	Chromatogram of Quercetin at 366 nm	162
5.30	Chromatogram of Rutin at 366 nm	163
5.31	Chromatogram of Stigma sterol at 366 nm	164
5.32	Chromatogram of Gallic acid at 366 nm	165
5.33	Chromatogram of Ellagic acid at 366 nm	166
5.34	Chromatogram of Catechin at 366 nm	167
5.35	Chromatogram of Epicatechin at 366 nm	168
5.36	Chromatogram of Piperine at 366 nm	169
5.37	Chromatogram of Polyherbal Formulation FA (f1) at 366 nm	170
5.38	Chromatogram of Polyherbal Formulation FB (f2) at 366 nm	171
5.39	Chromatogram of Polyherbal Formulation FC (f3) at 366 nm	172
5.40	Chromatogram of Polyherbal Formulation FD (f4) at 366 nm	173

5.41	Chromatogram of Polyherbal Formulation FE (f5) at 366 nm	174
5.42	Chromatogram of Polyherbal Formulation FF (f6) at 366 nm	175
5.43	TLC of Polyherbal Formulation FA, FB and FC at 254 nm	176
5.44	TLC of Polyherbal Formulation FA, FB and FC at 366 nm	176
5.45	TLC of FD (f4) at 366 nm	177
5.46	TLC of FE (f5) at 366 nm	177
5.47	TLC of FF (f6) at 366 nm	177
5.48	TLC of Polyherbal Formulations (FA,FB,FC,FD,FE,FF) with standards at 254 nm	178
5.49	TLC of Polyherbal Formulations (FA,FB,FC,FD and FF) with standards at 366 nm	178
5.50	Chromatogram of Quercetin, Rutin and Stigma sterol at 420 nm	181
5.51	Chromatogram of Gallic acid, Ellagic acid, Catechin and Epicatechin at 420 nm	182
5.52	Chromatogram of Piperine, Polyherbal FA (f1), FB (f2) and FC (f3) at 420 nm	183
5.53	Chromatogram of Polyherbal FD (f4), FE (f5) and FF (f6) at 420 nm	184
5.54	Peak list of Standards and Polyherbal Formulations at 420 nm	187
5.55	Chromatogram of Quercetin at 420 nm	188
5.56	Chromatogram of Rutin at 420 nm	189
5.57	Chromatogram of Stigma sterol at 420 nm	190
5.58	Chromatogram of Gallic acid at 420 nm	191
5.59	Chromatogram of Ellagic acid at 420 nm	192
5.60	Chromatogram of Catechin acid at 420 nm	193
5.61	Chromatogram of Epicatechin acid at 420 nm	194
5.62	Chromatogram of Piperine acid at 420 nm	195
5.63	Chromatogram of Polyherbal formulation FA (f1) at 420 nm	196
5.64	Chromatogram of Polyherbal formulation FB (f2) at 420 nm	197
5.65	Chromatogram of Polyherbal formulation FC (f3) at 420 nm	198
5.66	Chromatogram of Polyherbal formulation FD (f4) at 420 nm	199

5.67	Chromatogram of Polyherbal formulation FE (f5) at 420 nm	200
5.68	Chromatogram of Polyherbal formulation FF (f6) at 420 nm	201
5.69	TLC of Polyherbal Formulations with Standards at 420 nm	202

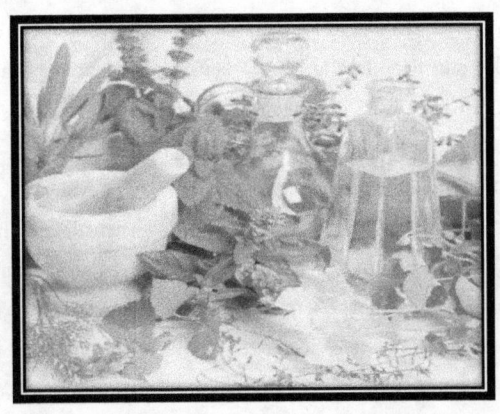

CHAPTER-1

Introduction

Chapter 1　　　　　　　　　　　　　　　　　　　　　　　　　　　　　　Introduction

1.1 Background: WHO (1999) defined as an endocrine disorder which reflected the inappropriate regulation of carbohydrate, lipid and protein metabolism in body. This results primarily in increasing blood glucose levels. If this variance and imbalanced condition does not revert back to normal and staying for a prolonged period of time, it develops hyperglycemia and in the long run leads to a syndrome called **diabetes mellitus**. Leonid (2009) and Ripoll et al (2011) depicted in their publications that In Egyptian manuscript from 1500 BCE diabetes was described as the first disease and mentioning it "too great emptying of urine". "Diabetes derived from the Greek word "**Diab**" was first used in 230 BCE (meaning to pass through, referring to cycle of heavy thirst and frequent urination); "mellitus" is the Latin word for "sweetened with honey which refers to presence of sugar in the urine. The disease was believed as uncommon during the time of Roman Empire with Galen who termed the disease "diarrhea of the urine".

Historical books reveals that since 200 BC diabetes mellitus was well known and identified disease in India and characterized in two types: a genetically based disorder and dietary related disorders i.e. Type 1 and Type 2 diabetes were recognized as separate conditions for the first time by the India physicians *Sushruta* and *Charaka* in 400-500 BCE. Diabetes Wikipedia and Ahmed A.M (2002) mentioned that many approaches were tried but useful, safe and effective treatment was not identified until the early part of the 20th century when Canadians Frederick Banting and Charles Herbert Best developed Insulin in 1921 and 1922.This was followed by development of long acting insulin NPH in the 1940s.

Many measures were tried since 1940 and numerous synthetic drugs were developed for the treatment of diabetes mellitus but the safe and effective treatment paradigm is yet to be achieved. International Federation has estimated that numbers of peoples with diabetes in 2003 was 194 million and forecasted that number may increase to 334 million by 2025.India leads the world with largest number of diabetic subjects earning the dubious distinction of being termed the "diabetes hub of the world" It is becoming the third "Killer" of the health of mankind after cancer and cardiac diseases. Dr Wild (2004) in Diabetes Care stated the global prevalence of diabetes. Dr. Wild investigation results indicated the occurrence of diabetes globally for all age-groups was likely to be 2.8% in 2000 and 4.4%

in 2030. The number of people with diabetes is anticipated to increase from 171 million in 2000 to 366 million in 2030. The occurrence of diabetes is greater in men than women however it is observed that there are more women with diabetes than men. The metropolitan population in developing countries is expected to be double between 2000 and 2030. The most important demographic change to diabetes dominance throughout the world appears to be the increase in the proportion of people >65 years of age. It is mentioned in IDF Diabetes Atlas that around 415 million people are suffered from diabetes worldwide in 2015. Figure 1.1 and 1.2 indicates the list of countries with highest number of diabetes patients estimated and projected in 2015 and 2030. It clearly indicates that India is moving forward to achieve the first ranking globally projected with greatest number of diabetes people in world in 2030. Mohan et al (2007) studies demonstrates the distribution of diabetes peoples in different parts of India, In 2001 prevalence of diabetes was higher in Hyderabad with 16.6% of diabetes people in the city. Thiruvanthipuram and Chennai accorded the 2nd and 3rd Position period of 1999 and 2001. Figure 1.3 highlighted that In India mostly southern part were in gripped of diabetes from 1999 to 2003, it could be because of south Indian people lifestyle and eating habits include mostly high calorie diet.

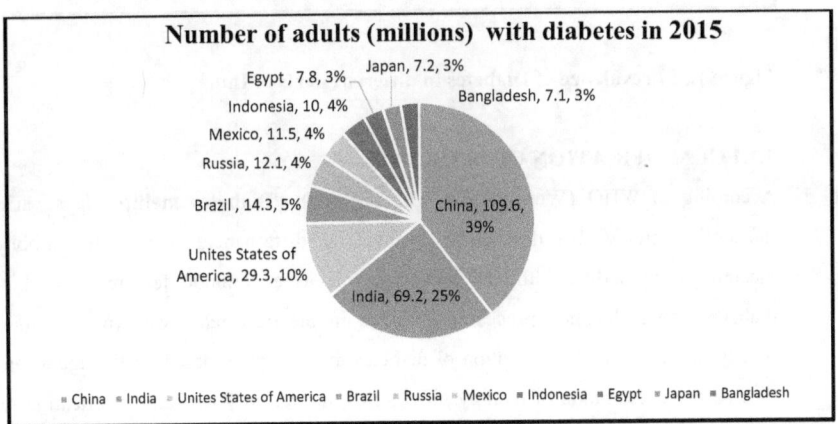

Figure.1.1: Countries with higher number of Diabetes subjects in year 2015

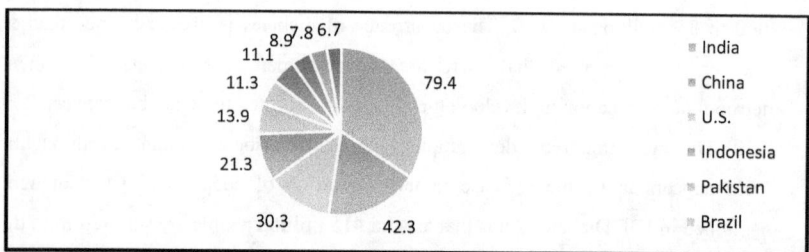

Figure.1.2: Countries with higher number of Diabetes subjects in year 2030

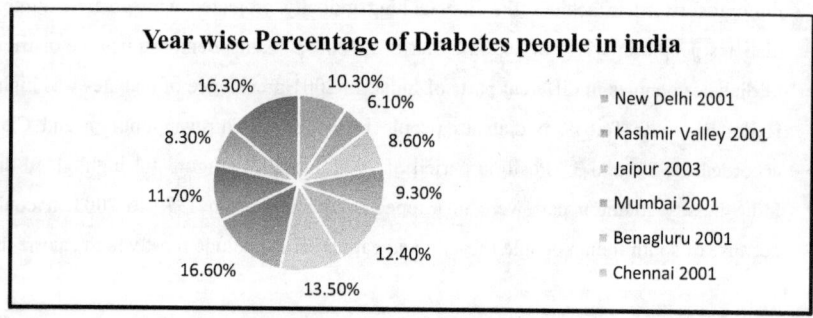

Figure.1.3: Prevalence of Diabetes in different parts of India

1.1.1 CLASSIFICATION OF DIABETES:

According to WHO (World Health Organization), "**Diabetes mellitus** is a variegated metabolic chronic disorder which resulted in disturbance of protein, carbohydrate metabolism in body". Although hyperglycemia as a common feature in all kinds of diabetes, the pathogenic processes involved in the occurrence of hyperglycemia vary widely, the previous classification of diabetes mellitus were based on the age at onset of disease or on the mode of therapy; in contrast, the recently revised classification reflects our greater understanding of the pathogenesis of each variant.

Chapter 1 — Introduction

Previous Classification:

Mayfield (1998) documented in their review that in 1979, the National Diabetes Data Group (NDDG) released a document arranging the nomenclature and definitions for diabetes mellitus

Diabetes mellitus can be classified in two types; two names were given according to clinical presentation.

1. "Insulin – dépendant diabètes mellites" (IDDM).
2. "Non-insulin-dépendent diabètes mellites" (NIDDM).

The discovery of other types of diabetes with specific pathophysiology did not framed into this classification system, to overcome this difficultynew classification has been provided along with mechanism of diabetes mellitus.

Revised classification:

It has been discussed in literature by Mayfield Jennifer (1998): In June 1997, an international expert committee of WHO issued a report with new approvals for the classification and diagnosis of diabetes mellitus

American Diabetes Association (2009) describes the Etiological Classification of Diabetesmellitus.

I. *Type 1 diabetes* (β-cell destruction, resulting in insulin deficiency)

A. Immune mediated
B. Idiopathic

II. *Type 2 diabetes* (may range mainly frominsulin resistance with comparative insulin deficiency and mainly to secretary defect with insulin resistance)

III. *Other peculiar different types*

A Genetic defect of β-cell function

1) Chromosome 12, HNF-1α (MODY3)
2) Chromosome 7, Glucokinase(MODY2)
3) Chromosome 20, HNF-4α(MODY1)
4) Chromosome 13, insulin promoter
5) Chromosome 17, HNF-1β(MODY5)
6) Chromosome 2, *NeuroD1* (MODY6)
7) Mitochondrial DNA
8) Others

B Genetic deficiencies in insulin deed
1) Type A insulin resistance diabetes
2) Rabson-Mendenhall syndrome
3) Lipoatrophic diabetes
4) Others

C Exocrine pancreas diseases
1 Pancreatitis
2. Trauma/pancreatectomy
3. Neoplasia
4. Cystic fibrosis
5. Hemochromatosis
6. Fibrocalculous pancreatopathy
7. Others

D. Endocrinopathies
1. Acromegaly
2. Cushing's syndrome
3. Glucagonoma
4. Pheochromocytoma
5. Hyperthyroidism
6. Somatostatinoma
7. Aldosteronoma
8. Others

E. Drug- or chemical-induced
1. Vacor
2. Pentamide
3. Nicotinic acid
4. Glucocorticoids
5. Thyroid hormone
6. Diazoxide
7. β - adrenergic agonists
8. Thiazides
9. Dilantin
10. α–Interferon

F. Infections
1. Congenital rubella
2. Cytomegalovirus
3. Others

G. Uncommon forms of immune mediate diabetes
1. "Stiff-man" syndrome
2. Anti-insulin receptor antibodies.
3. Others

IV. *Gestational diabètes mellites (GDM)*

Type 1 Diabètes mellites

It is reported that with every hour of day, someone is identified with type 1 diabetes, which every year number increases for more than $100 billion in health care budgets in the U.S. alone. Usually after passing the age of 30, Type 1 diabetes makes heavy gripped on people. These people not only became dependent on insulin for life but also get suffered from the risk of blindness, cardiac disease and kidney failure is a prevalent threat. Insulin is only used as a life support and cannot be used to eliminate the diabetes. (Diabetes Wikipedia).

Type 1 diabetes is harmful to both the children and to childhood. it can be controlled by eating carefully selected diet, by checking blood glucose level each day on every 2nd or 3rd hr. (by lancing a finger).It requires a daily vigilance and strict rules in life. It means all families will have to live by a clock, day and night with an average of 15 yrs. less than normal. Type 1 Diabetes is a disorder characterized by damage of the insulin-producing β-cells of the pancreas and person totally become dependent on insulin injection on daily basis.

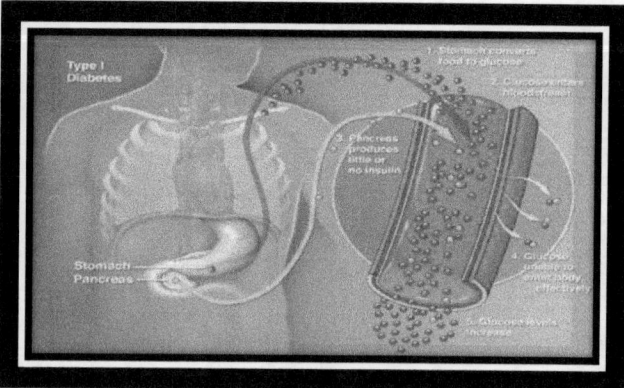

Figure 1.4: Type 1 Diabetes mellitus

This type of diabetes extends over the large area of North America and Europe, but the percentage of disease proliferation varies by geographical location. The disease can also affect adults, but majority of cases have been reported from the children that's why it has traditionally been called as "juvenile diabetes". It is an autoimmune disorder which is caused by a loss of beta cells of pancreas along with the release of directed against insulin and islet cell. The primary treatment for type 1 diabetes is only the replacement of insulin which can be started even from the initial stage of occurrence of disease. The deficiency of insulin can develop diabetic ketoacidosis.

Mary Tyler Moore, the chairman of JDRF, (Juvenile Diabetes Research Foundation) has said, **"Diabetes is just like time bomb which can go off today, tomorrow, next year, or ten years from now—a time bomb affecting millions...one which must be defused".** The only resolution is to treat the disease since earliest stage. That's why the organization is having only mission to find out the treatment for this disease and its complications through the support of research as soon as possible.

Type 2 Diabetes mellitus

A condition which can be characterized by high blood glucose levels due to a jumble of malfunctioning of insulin and imperfect sensitivity to insulin (often termed reduced insulin sensitivity). In early stages mainly, the sensitivity of insulin decreases. So increase in plasma glucose level can be upturned by using the recover insulin sensitivity or decreases glucose production by the liver, but with the passage of time imbalance of insulin secretion worsens and therapeutic replacement of insulin often becomes essential. This type of diabetes is common and it is expected that it affects the 90 % of population worldwide. "National Institute of Diabetes and Digestive and Kidney Disease" also explained the relationship between Type 2 disease with and aging. Although in the last years it has gradually more affected the older children and young people. Therefore, this type of diabetes was named as an *adult-onset diabetes* or *maturity-onset diabetes*.

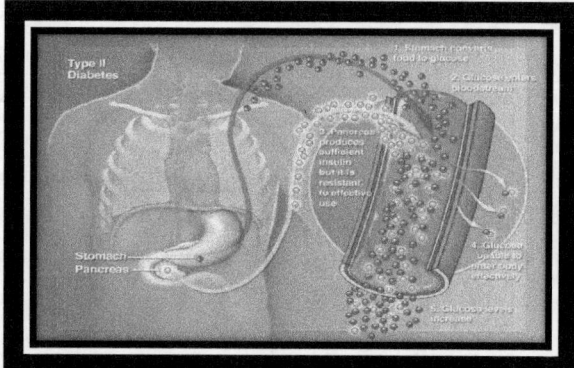

Figure 1.5: Type 2 Diabetes mellitus

Other specific types are currently less common causes of diabetes mellitus and can be identified in specific manner. These types of diabetes do not fit into type-1, type-2, or gestational diabetes. The cause of others types of diabetes may be specific genetic conditions (such as maturity-onset diabetes of youth), malnutrition, drugs, infections, surgery and other illnesses. Nichols Hannah and Bay nest HW (2015)

Gestational Diabetes
A condition characterized by high blood glucose level due to the insufficient insulin secretion and imperfect insulin responsiveness. It resembles to type-2 diabetes in several respects. It develops in women during pregnancy. Generally, this type of diabetes disappears in women after the birth of child. Women with Gestational Diabetes usually are at risk for developing type-2 diabetes later on in life. Baynest HW (2015). So, it is important that women should take care of blood glucose level throughout the life and should be careful initially to normalize maternal blood levels to avoid complications in the infant.

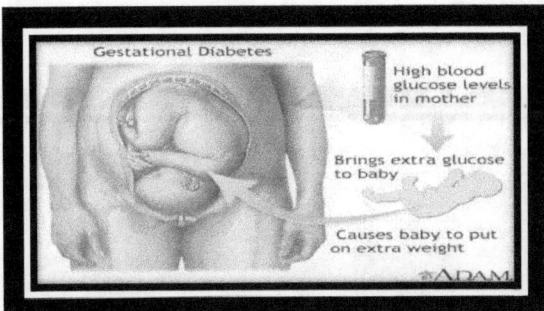

Figure 1.6: Gestational diabètes

Latent Auto-immune Diabètes in Adults

Latent autoimmune diabetes in adults (LADA) is a hereditary genetically linked disorder in which body recognizes the pancreas as a foreign element and destroys the beta cells of pancreas that is the source of insulin. Simply it can be stated as an autoimmune disorder, including LADA, is an "allergy to self."

It has been reported by Stenström et al (2005) that in initial stages LADA typically presents as type-2 diabetes and due to this it is sometimes not correctly diagnosed as such. However, LADA closely resembles to type-1 diabetes and shares common physiological features of type 1 for upset metabolism, genetics factors and autoimmune features, however children are not affected by LADA and are classified distinctly as being separate from juvenile diabetes.

1.1.2 SYMPTOMS OF Diabetes: Below figure is self-explanatory and gives the common symptoms of diabetes.

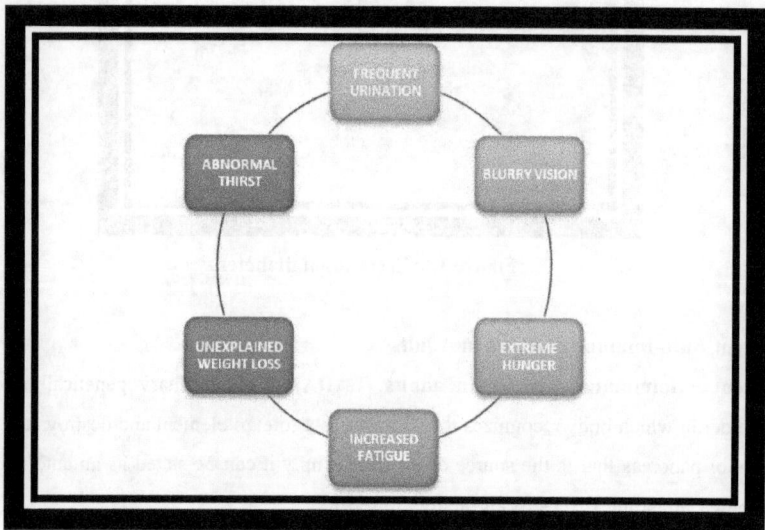

Figure 1.7: Symptoms of Diabetes

1.2 Ayurvedic approach in managing the diabetes mellitus

1.2.1 Introduction:

Krishna K et al (2013) described the Ayurveda as the ancient Indian system of medicine, also known as "Science of life" is originated from the word "**Ayu**" (life) and "**Veda**" (knowledge) and is supposed to have originated from fourth Veda i.e. Athar Veda. It has got 8 branches (Ashtang Ayurveda which include Shalya (surgery), Shalakya(ENT, ophthalmology,dentistry)Kaychikitsa(Medicine),Bhutavidya(Dermatology),KaumaryaBhritya (Paediatrics), Rasayantantra (Rejuvenation),Agattantra (Toxicology),Bajikaran (Geriatrics).

According to Ayurveda, all living and nonliving things are made up of Panchmahabhoot (5 basic elements) namely Prithvi (earth), Jal (water), Vayu (air), Agni (fire), Akash (ether).In human body the structural part and all hollow spaces like abdominal and chest cavities are represented by Prithvi and Akash respectively.

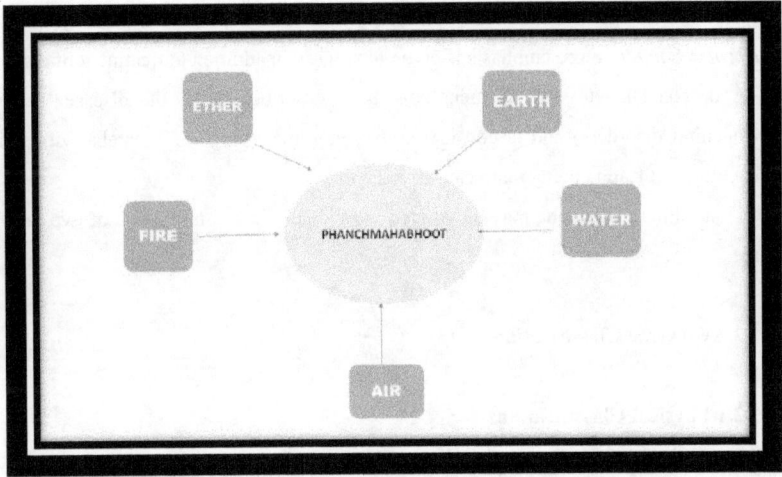

Figure 1.8: Panch-mahabhoot (5 elements)

Therefore all the biological, psychological and pathophysiological functions are governed by air, fire and water elements for which Ayurvedic terminology of Vata, Pitta and Kapha has been given. Individually they are called "Doshas" and their combinations as three Dosha.They remain in balanced state and provide health. Any vikriti (Imbalance) in above state may lead to disease and ailments. They are also manifested by above 5 elements (Panchmahabhoot) and according to predominance of elements.Vata is composed of Vayu (air) and Akash (ether),Pitta of agni(fire) and Jal(water) and Kapha is a combination of jal(water)andprithvi(earth)Summary of basic principles of Ayurveda that illustrates relationship between Panchmahabhoot, tridosha, rasa and gunas.

The Ayurvedic treatment is directed towards restoration of imbalanced state of Vata, Pitta and Kapha by meticulous use of drugs of plants, animals and minerals origin as they are also made up of Panchmahabhoot.

Earliest treaties of Ayurveda are *Charak Samhita* and *Sushruta Samhita* which dates back to 2500 BC and 500 BC respectively.*Charak Samhita* deals with medicine covering basic principles, etiology and treatment of diseases besides methods for healthy living; In *Sushratra Samhita* more emphasis is given to surgery in addition to treatment of diseases.

In Ayurveda Diabetes (Madhumeha) has been described under the disease 'Premeha' (uriogenital disorders) and is considered as penultimate stage of Premeha with vitiated Vata,Pitta and Kapha being main causative factor.

The Vata, Pitta and Kapha may be vitiated individually in a combination of two or all the three.

1.2.2 Ayurvedic Classification

1.2.2.1 Physical Classifications

Prameha (diabetes) can be divided in two types:

1) *Apatharpanauthaja prameha* depicting the slender/lean diabetic.
2) *Santharpanauthaja prameha* linked with obese diabetic.

Anetiological classification of diabetic patients

1) *Sahaja prameha* (congenital)
2) *Apathyanimittaja prameha* (due to bad eating and unhealthy life style)

The symptoms of onset of *Premeha* as described in diabetes cure in Ayurveda are as under:
- Sweda   :   Excessive sweating
- Ang-gand   :   Foul smell in body
- Shithil-Ang   :   Looseness of body

Chapter 1   *Introduction*

- Shaiya-asanasukh : Desire to sit or lay down
- Hridayapadeh : Heaviness in chest
- Netropadeha : Heaviness in eye
- Jivha-padeha : Feeling of coated tongue
- Shravanopadeha : Feeling of coating in ear
- Ghana-ang : Heaviness of body
- Kesh-vridhi : Excessive growth of hair
- Nakhvridhi : Excessive growth of nails
- Sheet-priya : Affinity towards cold
- Gala-shosh : Dry and cold throat
- Talushosh : Dryness of palate
- Mukh-madhaurya : Sweetness in month
- Kar-dah : Burning sensation in palm
- Pad-dah : Burning sensation in foot
- Motra-madhurya : Sweetness in urine

Kaphaja: Symptoms of *Kaphaj* Diabetes available at www.diabetesneed.com

- *Avipakam* - indigestion
- *Aruchi* - Loss of appetite
- *Chardi* - Vomiting tendency
- *Athinidra* - Excessive sleep
- *Kasam* - Cough
- *Peenasam* - Cold with running nose

***Pittaja*: Symptoms of *Pittaj* diabetes**

- *Vasthimehanyotoda* - Pain in Bladder & urinary tract
- *Mushkavatharanam* - Pain in testes

- *Jwara* - Fever
- *Daham* - Burning sensation
- *Trishna* - Thirst
- *Amlika* - Acidity
- *Moorcha* - Giddiness
- *Vitbhedanam* - Loose Motion
- *Hridayashoola* - Pain in heart region
- *Nidranasam* - Loss of sleep

Vathaja:Symptoms of *Vataj* diabetes

- *Udavartham* - Upward movement of *vatha*.
- *Kambam* - Tremor
- *Hridgraham* - Gripping pain in chest region
- *Lolatha* - Affinity
- *Soolam* - Pain
- *Anidratha* - Insomnia
- *Sosha* - Wasting
- *Kasam* - Cough
- *Swasam* - Difficulty to breath
- *Badhapureeshathwa* - Constipation

1.2.2.2 *Charak Samhita* has classified diabetes into three types: *Charaka*.

1. **Sadhya** - Curable
2. **Yapya** - Palliable
3. **Asadhya** - Incurable

<u>Sadhya</u>: Under this category patients have been diagnosed very first in the onset of *Prameha*. The patients who are *sthoola* [obese] comes under this category and the origin of disease is due *apathyaja* [poor living habits].

Yapya: Under this category Patients have *Pittaja* prameha and certain types of *kaphaja Prameha*. However, *Yapya* {palliable} the disease can be controlled with treatment.

Asadhya: define the incorrigible form of prameha and inherited diabetes. Patients suffering from this variety are *Krisha* {lean}.

Ayurvedic practitioners address diet modifications suggest drugs and exercise when working with people suffering from diabetes. Removing sugar and emphasizing complex carbohydrates is a first line of defense for both Ayurvedic and Western understanding. As diabetes is a disease of the digestive system, it is important to know that in Ayurvedic philosophy, digestion is believed to occur in three stages. The first is Kaphic in nature occurring in the mouth and stomach where water and earth elements are extracted from the food. Next is a pitta (bile) stage, with acids in the stomach and alkali in small intestine extracting the fire element. Finally, in the vatta (wind) phase, the air and either element is extracted in the large intestine. Therefore, Ayurvedic treatises like Charaka and Sushruta Samhitas have included special chapters on Ayurvedic preparations of nutrients and herbs which can aid in the re-balancing at different stages during digestion. In literature Sharma et al (2011) illustrated that Ayurvedic preparations are made mainly on the thoughts of *Rasa* (taste), *Guna* (qualitative attributes), *Veerya* (therapeutic effect) and *Vipaka* (over all post-digestive effect of a medicine). When the above principle does not work then ayurveda proposes the principle of *Prabhav* mean unpredictable action of a drug. Such materials were meticulously studied by the ancient stages, based on the **Prakriti Sama Samavayarabdha** (predictable) principle and those not falling in to this category are classified under ***Vikriti Vishama Samavayarabdha*** which means unpredictable action, not consistent with *Ras,Guna,Virya* and *Vipak*. As a result, **Ayurvedic discipline of drug action on human body has become sacrosanct allowing only additions, but no deletions.**

Parasuraman et al 2014 mentioned that herbal drugs formulated in Ayurveda on two ways:

A. Formulated as single drug.

B. Formulated in combination of two or more than two drugs.

When two or more herbs are mixed in formulations, they are called as polyherbal formulations. The idea of polyherbalism is peculiar although it is difficult to explain in term of modern parameters while *Sarangdhar Samhita* another treaty of Ayurveda highlights the thoughts of synergism and antagonism behind **Polyherbal formulations**

1.2.3 Overview on Marketed Ayurvedic Herbal Medicine

Earlier, the Ayurvedic physicians (Vaidya's) prepare their own medicine for the treatment of patients but on account of heavy demand for commercial manufacturing of Ayurvedic drugs, without compromising with the basic principles of Ayurveda, has started under the license from Drug Control Authorities and manufacturing is done as per the guidelines of Drug and Cosmetics act of Government of India.

Modak et al (2007) gatheredthe commercially available Ayurvedic preparations in their review, as per their analysis number of Ayurvedic drugs for the treatment of diabetes is available in the market and some of them are:

Diabecon

Manufactured By: *Himalaya*

Chemical ingredients: *Gymnema sylvestre, Pterocarpus marsupium, Glycyrrhiza glabra, Casearia esculenta, Syzygium cumini, Asparagus racemosus, Boerhavia diffusa, Sphaeranthus indicus, Tinospora cordifolia, Swertia chirata, Tribulus terrestris, Phyllanthus amarus, Gmelina arborea, Gossypium herbaceum, Berberis aristata, Aloe vera, Triphala, Commiphora wightii, shilajeet, Momordica charantia, Piper nigrum, Ocimum sanctum, Abutilon indicum, Curcuma longa, Rumex maritimus*

Dose: Recommended to be taken 2 tablets twice or thrice daily 30 minutes before meals on an empty stomach

Actions:

It increases the consumption of glucose and support the restoration of beta cell. It put forth action by reducing the glycated hemoglobin levels and controls the albumin urea and lipid profile. It also helps in reduction of long term diabetic complications.

When Diabecon is used as an adjuvant in IDDM and NIDDM, it is recommended to titrate the dose of insulin and oral anti-diabetic under the supervision of a health professional.

The **clinical study** of diabecon revealed that out of thirty NIDDM patients, all showed a significant reduction in sugar and glycosylated hemoglobin levels after taking Diabecon. Out of 15 patients with diabetes were taking high doses of OHA. Diabecon was also shown to be effective even when used with other OHA's in NIDDM treatment.

Epinsulin

Manufactured By: Swastik formulations.

Chemical Composition: Vijaysar (*Pterocarpus marsupium*)

Dose: Recommended to be taken 2 tablets daily before meals

Actions:

It contains Epicatechin as main active ingredient. Epicatechin is benzopyran molecule.

It increases the cAMP of beta cells of pancreatic islets which help in increased in insulin release. It facilitates the transformation of proinsulin to insulin by growing cathepsin activity. It inhibited the Na/K ATPase activity from patient's erythrocytes. It regulates disturbed metabolism of glucose and lipids. It continues the integrity of all organ systems affected by the disease. It is depicted to be a beneficial for Non-Insulin Dependent Diabetes Mellitus (NIDDM) and a good adjuvant for Insulin Dependent Diabetes Mellitus (IDDM), in order to reduce the amount of desired insulin. It is advised to be taken along with present oral hypoglycemic drugs and is known to prevent diabetic complication. It has good hypoglycemic activity

Pancreatic Tonic: Ayurvedic herbal supplement: It is a botanical mixture of Ayurvedic herbs and is currently available in market.

Bitter gourd powder

Marketed by: Garry and Sun.

Chemical Composition: Momrdica Charantia

Dose: 1 teaspoon daily empty stomach in the morning.

Actions:

It decreases the blood sugar and urine sugar level. It purifies the blood and also increases the immunity of the body to fight against the infections. Bitter Gourd has amazing therapeutic and medicinal values. It has an exceptional antidiabetic activity. Many Phytoconstituents like saponins, alkaloids, reducing sugars, bitter glycosides, phenolics, oils, free acids, polypeptides and steroids are present in Bitter gourd. It has been reported that bitter gourd powder has hypoglycemic activity in addition to

Stomachic, astringent, hepatic stimulant, emmenagogue, anthelmintic and blood purifier actions.

Clinical study of *Momordica charantia* fruit extract in 9 patients with diabetes mellitus showed significant decrease in fasting blood glucose levels. The onset of action was similar to that of standard insulin.

Dia-Care

Manufactured By: *Admark Herbals Ltd.*

Dose and method of application: Recommended to take 5 gms. (approx. 1 tea spoon) powder, mix it with 1 glass of water (Approx. 200 ml.) stir it properly and kept it overnight. Drink the water on empty stomach in the morning leaving the powder at the bottom of the glass. (20-30 minutes after drink, tea, coffee or breakfast can be taken.) Add ½ glass fresh water to same glass and mix it again, leave it all day till evening and drink only water. Half an hour before dinner, (leaving the powder at bottom of glass). Discard the sediment and take fresh medicine for next day.

Chemical Composition: *Cressa Cretica*-10 %, *Vitex negundo*-10%, *Terminatia Chebula*-10 %, *Elugenia Jamboloma*-10%, *Picrorhiza Kurroa*-20 %, *Enicostama Littorale*-20%, *Azadirachta Indicas* -20 %

Actions:

It is useful and effective for both Type 1 and Type 2 diabetes. Patients taking insulin get eventually released from the dependency on it. The whole treatment completed in 6 phases, each phase is of 90 days and approximately within 18 months diabetes can be controlled.

Diabetes-Daily Care

Chemical composition: Diabetes-Daily Care containing Alpha Lipoic Acid, Cinnamon 4% Extract, Chromax, Vanadium, Fenugreek 50% extract, *Gymnema sylvestre* 25% extract, Momordica 7% extract, Licorice Root 20% extract

Dose: Recommended to be taken 1 capsule three times per day

Manufactured By: *Nature's Health Supply*

Actions:

It is a distinctive, natural medicine, effective in maintaining the sugar metabolism. Diabetes Daily Care™ was mainly developed for type 2 diabetics and consists of all-natural components in the optimum proportion for human use.

Gurmar powder

Manufacturing By: *Garry and Sun*

Chemical Composition: *Gymnema sylvestre*

Actions:

Gurmar is known for its antidiabetic activity. It stimulates the insulin secretion and helps in decreasing the glucose level in blood. It is reported to be good in regulating the metabolic activities of kidney and liver. In diabetes when it put on tongue it gives bitter taste by blocking the sweet taste receptors. It also acts as diuretic and cardiac stimulant.

One of the Clinical trial report of *Gymnema sylvestre* published in 1992 carried out on 16 healthy volunteers and 43 subjects with Type 2 diabetic patients. 16 healthy volunteers received *gymnema* only and 43 Type 2 diabetic patients received either *gymnema* or tolbutamide for 21 days. In this study subjects were not assigned to any groups and study was not blinded. On 7th day the non-diabetic patients experienced a significant reduction in fasting blood sugar (FBS, from 80.8 mg/dL to 71.6 mg/dL). The diabetic patients in the *gymnema* treated arm experienced significant reductions in both FBS (152 mg/dL to 133 mg/dL) and post-prandial blood sugar (PPBS, 215 mg/dL to 142 mg/dL) at 21 days. The diabetic patients in the tolbutamide treatment arm also showed significant reductions in both FBS and PPBS at day 7th, but not at day 14th. Total cholesterol level were also reported to be decreased. P values were not provided for this short, non-randomized study.

Diabeta

Manufactured By*: Ayurvedic Cure*

Chemical composition: *Gymnema sylvestre*, *Vinca rosea* (Periwinkle), *Curcuma longa* (Turmeric), *Azadirachta indica* (Neem), *Pterocarpus marsupium* (Kino Tree), *Momordica charantia* (Bitter Gourd), *Syzygium cumini* (Black Plum), *Acacia arabica* (Black Babhul), *Tinospora cordfolia* , *Zingiber officinale* (Ginger)

Dose: Suggested dosage is 1 – 2 capsules a day or as prescribed by the doctor.

Actions:

It is very effective anti-diabetic formulation with combination of effective immunomodulatory, anti-stress, hepatoprotective agents and anti-hyperlipidemic agents. Diabeta control the blood glucose level by acting on different sites by different ways. It is safe and effective in treatment of Diabetes Mellitus as a single agent supplement. "Diabeta" confers a sense of well -being in patients and provides the symptomatic relief of complaints like weakness, pain in legs, giddiness, body ache, polyuria and pruritus.

Clinical studies have showed a very low point of disulfiram-like effect in patients, who were taking Diabeta capsules. Studies conducted on normal subjects (single dose study) with Diabeta showed absorption in an hour while peak drug levels are at 4 hours.

Syndrex

Manufactured By*: Plethico Laboratory*

Chemical composition: germinated fenugreek seed

Dose: Suggested to be taken 1-2 capsules in day.

Actions: In the last 1000 years fenugreek is used as an ingredient in traditional formulations. Researchers are going on to find the mechanism of action of fenugreek as an antidiabetic drug. Research investigations have showed that treatment with Syndrex increased the activity of antioxidant enzymes catalase, glutathione reductase and superoxide dismutase

It may be seen that many plants have been used individually or in combinations for treatment of diabetes and its complications. One of the major problems with herbal formulations is that the active ingredients are not well defined with mechanism of action. It is important to identify the active component and their molecular interaction, which could help to analyze therapeutic efficacy of the product and also to standardize the product. Researchers are now pushing their efforts to investigate mechanism of action of some of these plants using model systems.

1.3. Need for investigation

Diabetes is one of foremost reason of increasing death next to cancer and heart diseases this is for the reason that outcome of hyperglycemia resulted many other complications in individuals and people becomes more prone to kidney failure, loss of vision, arthritis, heart diseases. Several medicines are available in the market for the treatment of diabetes, in spite of the availability of these medicines diabetes creates havoc in society and maintaining its ranking in causing death in world. Many allopathic medicines are also available in the world for treating diabetes but now people are looking forward to other alternative therapies i.e. herbal therapies and have putting trust on these herbal medicines as these medicines provides less side effects and greater effectiveness. Therefore, research for investigation on herbal plants to explore the effective herbal formula on the Ayurvedic principles is of great interest and will keep on developing the interest in scholars unless the researcher and science combination could come up with the most potential standardized herbal drug with no side effects. Even though single herb formulation has been well established due to their active phytoconstituent's, usually present in minute amount and sometimes they are insufficient to achieve the desirable therapeutic effects. Scientific studies have revealed that these plants of varying potency when combined may theoretically produce a greater result, as compared to individual use of the plant and also the sum of their individual effect, thus positive herb-herb interaction produce synergism, which could be pharmacokinetic synergism or pharmacodynamic synergism. Due to the presence of multiple components in the herbal products, the effects arising from herb-herb or herb-drug interactions are often unpredictable and complicated. Various types of pharmacokinetic and pharmacogenomics interactions from herb-drug combinations have been well described and documented in recent literature. On the other hand, much less information is available on herb-herb interaction, although herb-herb combination has been used and documented as a desirable therapeutic approach in China since the time of the Yellow Emperor's Canon of Internal Medicine (Huangdi Neijing) more than 2,000 years ago.

"One drug, one target, one disease" method continued as traditional typical pharmaceutical approach to the development of medicines and treatment strategies. However, over the last decade, this mono-substance therapy model has gradually shifted toward the adoption of combination therapies, in which multiple active components are employed. It is believed that herbal formulations with multicomponent can give better and effective results as an antidiabetic agent as compare to single herbal drug. Recent evidence from Devita et al.(1975), Chesney et al.(2000), Jukema and van der Hoorn, (2004).has demonstrated that combination therapy could provide greater therapeutic benefits to diseases such as diabetes, cancer and AIDS, all of which involved complicated etiology and pathophysiology and therefore are difficult to treat using single drug target approach.

Scientific studies have been proved that plants molecule in combination could give better therapeutic effects as compare to single plants may be because of its positive herb interactions. This is called synergism in which effect of one drug is potentiated by effect of another drug used in combination. One of the survey done by Xian Zhou et al (2016) justified the synergistic effects of multicomponent and described the detailed definition of synergy which means the interaction of two or more agents to produce a combined effect greater than the sum of their individual effects. Additionally, Spinella M (2002) described the concept of synergism is mainly based on two modes of action 1) Pharmacodynamics and 2) Pharmacokinetics synergism. The first type of synergy describes two or more agents that work on the same receptors or biological targets result in enhanced therapeutic outcomes through their positive interactions. The second type of synergy results from interactions between two or more agents during their pharmacokinetic processes (absorption, distribution, metabolism and elimination) leading to changes of the agents quantitatively in the body and hence their therapeutic effects.

Chun-Tao Che et al (2013) wonderfully explained herb herb combination for positive therapeutic enhancement in their review article. This review strongly highlights the available scientific and clinical evidence to supports the combined use of herbs. The desirable effects are those which can provide the additional therapeutic benefit as expected outcome of combination therapy. When the herbs used in combination the effects can be complicated since various individual components interact with each other in combination.

The concept of herb-herb interaction, based on the beliefs of positive or negative outcomes, was therefore developed. It was realized that the presence of one herb may alter the effect of the other when they are co-administered. The combined effect, either complementary or antagonistic, would be manifested in the clinical outcome. For example, Xie, Z (2000) reported in their research that the Decoction of Ephedra (Mahuang Tang), which contains ephedra, cinnamon twig, bitter apricot seed, and licorice root. This prescription is used not only for its diaphoretic effect, but also for the relief of coughing and asthma, as well as reducing headaches and general aching during common cold. All of these symptoms are interpreted by the Chinese medicine theory to be caused by excessive "coldness" and "wind" in the body. The co-administration of multiple ingredients would result in complementary interactions to reduce symptoms of common cold or influence the illness. The scenario is comparable to the modern combination medicines with antipyretic, cough suppressant and nasal decongestant properties used in the treatment of common cold.

Liu RH (2004) and Spinella M (2002) reported that Cumin, black pepper and asafetida are used together traditionally to reduce bloating due to weak digestion; whereas guduchi and turmeric combination promotes one's immunity. So here we observed that effect is potentiated with the use of other plants added in polyherbal formula.

Literature reviews have shown that researchers developed the many Polyherbals with high effectiveness. Important of them are listed below

Dihar by Patel et al (2009)

Diabet by Umamaheswari et al (2009)

Diasol by Hamid BSSet al (2010)

Dianex by Mutalik et al (2005)

DRF/AY/5001 by Naik et al (2008)

Diabrid by Qadri et al (2011)

These all formulations are having good sign of antidiabetic property. It was found that these all Polyherbals were formulated with the extent use of traditional well known medicinal plants however there are some emerging plants like *Annona squamosa, Morus alba, Nelumbo nucifera,Psidium guajava* which also required to be exploited in terms of antidiabetic activity at extract level, molecular level. It was also expected that polyherbal combinations of these plants would also be effective and possess good accessibility and better affordability.

With this cumulative focus including the development of in-house standardization parameters, need for study was executed with the aim to develop new combination which could provide significant antidiabetic activity in animal model and can further provide the future aspects to exploited commercially and can be upgraded in any other dosage forms for clinical trial study.

CHAPTER-2

Aim and Objective

Of

Work

Chapter 2 — Aim and Objective of Work

Diabetes is dreadful disorder of this century. It is believed that by 2030 every 3rd person will be suffered from diabetes. Although several synthetic drugs are available in market for treatment of diabetes mellitus but with long use, these drugs could have develop the serious side effects. Adverse drug reactions are one of the main problems associated with the synthetic drugs. It is reported in USA that 10-25 % of patients experience adverse drug reaction which brings about to 7 % hospital admission. All these complications decrease the interest of mankind towards the use allopathic drugs. About 80% of People are now more inclined towards the use of herbal Ayurvedic drugs for the management of diabetes. Ayurveda an ancient Indian system of medicine with dates back to 2500 BC has described the etiology causative factors and treatments of diabetes mellitus (*Madumeh*). A number of traditionally used plant drugs like *Pterocarpus marsupium* (Vijaysar), *Gymnema sylvestre* (Gurmar), *Coccinia indica* (Kundru), *Momordica charantia* (Karela), *Piper longum* (Pippali), *Syzium cumini* (Jamun) have been effectively used either alone or in combination for the management of diabetes mellitus.

Latest research on plant drugs for antidiabetic activity has resulted in identification of potential antidiabetic drugs (emerging antidiabetic drugs); some of them commonly available in India are *Annona squamosa* (शरीफ़ा), *Morus alba* (शहतूत), *Nelumbo nucifera* (कमल), *Psidium guajava* (अमरूद).

Review of Literatures on all above identified plant drugs has revealed dose required for therapeutic activity (antidiabetic activity) along with their mode of actions like reduction in alpha amylase activity, absorption of carbohydrates from gastrointestinal tract (GIT), regeneration of pancreatic β-cells, increase in insulin sensitivity, reduction in alpha glucosidase activity, increase in serum insulin level.

Therefore, in present study it is proposed to develop the 6 formulations from extracts of above mentioned plant drugs in following manner:

Combination was done with reported therapeutic dose of drugs for antidiabetic activity in the above identified traditional and emerging plants drugs.

Plants drugs were combined in such way that one formulation should cover most of targeted sites of action to induce antidiabetic activity.

1) Formulation A consists of mixture of traditional antidiabetic and emerging antidiabetic plants drugs extracts wiz. *Annona squamosa, Morus alba, Coccinia india, Nelumbo nucifera, Gymnea sylvestre* with *Piper longum* (as bioavailability enhancer)
2) Formulation B consists of mixture of extracts of traditional and emerging plants drug extracts wiz. *Annona squamosa, Morus alba, Nelumbo nucifera, Syzium cumini* without *Piper longum*.
3) Formulation C consists of mixture of traditional antidiabetic and emerging antidiabetic plant drugs extracts wiz *Nelumbo nucifera, Psidium guajava, Gymnea sylvestre, Momordica charantia* and *Piper longum*.

Combination was done with fixed dose of drugs for antidiabetic activity in the above identified traditional and emerging plants drugs.

1) Formulation D consists of emerging antidiabetic plant drugs extracts wiz. *Annona squamosa, Morus alba, Nelumbo nucifera, Psidium guajava* with *Piper longum* (used as bioavailability enhancer) using fixed quantity of each drug.
2) Formulation E consists of traditionally used plants drugs extracts wiz. *Momordica charantia, Pterocarpus marsupium, Syzium cumini, Gymnea sylvestre* with *Piper longum* (used as bioavailability enhancer) using fixed quantity of extracts of each drug.

3) Formulation F consists of mixture traditional plants drugs and emerging plants drugs extract using fixed quantity of each drug.

These all six polyherbal formulation compared and investigated for antidiabetic activity with oral hypoglycemic agent Glibenclamide.

The complete methodology is divided in to 7 Phases:

Phase 1- Procurement and quality assessment of plant materials: Quality assessment and authentication of plant material (leaves) on the basis of different parameters like morphology, total ash value, alcohol extractive value etc. as given in Ayurvedic Pharmacopoeia of India and other Pharmacopoeias.

Phase 2 - Preparation of extracts and Preliminary Phytochemical screening of plant extracts with respect of group of compounds like alkaloids, glycosides, carbohydrates, terpenoids, steroids.

Phase 3- Design and Development of Polyherbal Formulations.

Phase 4- Acute toxicity study of polyherbal formulation as per OECD guidelines.

Phase 5–Oral glucose tolerance test of all formulations

Phase 6-Antidiabetic activity and assessment of following biochemical parameters:
a) Total Cholesterol(TC)
b) Total Triglycerides (TG)
c) High Density Lipoprotein (HDL)
d) Low Density Lipoprotein (LDL)
e) Urea
f) Creatinine

g) Serum Glutamate Oxaloacetic acid Transferase (SGOT)
h) Serum Glutamate Pyruvate Transferase (SGPT)

Results and Statistical analysis of pharmacological data by two-way ANOVA

Phase 7– Quality control/Standardization of Polyherbal formulations on the basis of following parameters:
a) Chromatographic analysis (TLC and HPTLC)
b) Heavy metal content determination
c) Microbial load determination

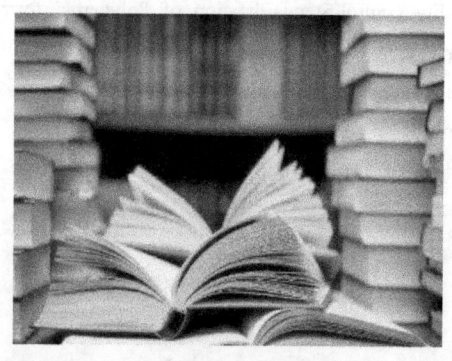

CHAPTER-3

Literature review

3.1 Diabetes: History and Treatment

3.1.1 History of diabetes

History of diabetes has been discussed by Ripoll *et al* (2011). It commenced from Egyptian manuscript from 1500 BC when it was first described as a disease which leads to urinate frequently. In 250 BCE the term "Diabetes mellitus" was first time used by Apollonius of Memphis. It is made up of two words i.e. "Diabetes" which is a Greek word (means: to pass through) and "mellitus "which is Latin word (means: sweet).Clinical description, symptoms of diabetes was first given by Greek physician Aretaeus Cappadocia. The first case observed was Type 1 Diabetes. Later on during the Middle Ages this disease was rarely mentioned. During the period of 980–1037 one of the Persian scientists Avicenna explained the detailed disease diabetes mellitus in "The canon of medicine". Avicenna was the first to describe diabetes insipidus very precisely. Types of Diabetes i.e. Type 1 and Type 2 was identified by *Charaka* and *Sushruta* in 400-500 CE.

It has been discussed by **Sarah et al (2004)** that as per the World Health Organization there are more than 180 million people worldwide suffering from diabetes and this number is likely to be double by 2030.As the year passes this disease has become widespread is increases worldwide, as of 2014 it is estimated that 387 million people have diabetes worldwide. Diabetes Voice (2014) estimated that in the year 2012-2014, diabetic related deaths are estimated to be 1.5 to 4.9 million per year. Diabetes and its complications therefore pose significant economic and public health consequences for individuals, families, health systems and countries.

3.1.2 Treatment of Diabetes mellitus

The intention in treating diabetes mellitus is to control the sugar level of blood. So individual life style, diet control and exercise play an important role in maintenance of sugar level in all types of diabetes. Type 1 Diabetes is treated with insulin therapy, exercise and diabetic diet while Type 2 Diabetes is treated with diabetic diet, exercise but if they are not sufficient to control the blood sugar level then oral medications are need to use.

3.1.2.1 Primary management of diabetes mellitus/Non-Pharmacological treatment

In literatures Clinton J. Choate (1998) and Kameswaran et al (2014) illustrated the conventional or non-pharmacological treatment of diabetes mellitus. Diabetes mellitus have been considered as dreadful lifestyle disorder. So Lifestyle improvement seems to be effective in the treatment of diabetes mellitus. By slightly changing lifestyle and focusing on diet, exercise and yoga anyone can control the adverse effect of diabetes and sugar level could be maintained. Kumar et al 2013 and ICMR guidelines for management of diabetes also stated the different curing aspects of diabetes by Yoga and described "YOGA" as rich heritage of Indian culture in management of not only diabetes but also in many diseases such as hypertension, thyroid disorders, rheumatoid arthritis and many more.

Diet: Dietary management is important for healthy life. The main aim of dietary management is to prevent the health complications related to diabetes, heart diseases by maintaining the body weight, blood glucose level, lipid profile. The dietary recommendations depend upon the individual's conditions so the food choice made by the individual should be ideal, regular and provide adequate nutrition for health and growth. Total calorie intake for diabetic person should not be more than 500 kcal per day.

Physical Activity: Exercise therapy is important and recommended for management of Type 1 and Type 2 diabetes. Physical activity combine with drug treatment can maintain the sugar level to optimum in person with type 2 diabetes. There are several benefit of regular exercise;

- Improvement in the glucose uptake by increasing insulin sensitivity
- Improves lipid profile, increasing HDL, reduces the triglycerides.
- Maintains body weight.
- Improves mental and physical well-being of individual
- Improves the quality of life.

Yoga: Yoga is science that can provide the therapeutic, preventive and protective effects in diabetes. It is an ancient science and is a form of exercise which involves different postures called asanas. Yoga is helpful in management of diabetes as practice of yoga improves the body and mind. It stimulates the different organs and glands and there by maintains the glandular secretions. It controls the blood sugar by increasing percentage insulin binding receptor in patients with type 2 diabetes. There are different types of asana which are effective in type 2 diabetes:

- Suryanamskar
- Bhastrika Pranayama
- Kapal- Bhati
- Tadasana
- Bhramari
- AnulomViloma
- Vajrasana
- Padmasana

Non-Pharmacological therapies can be considered as perfect epitome in controlling the blood sugar level in diabetes mellitus. It ensured the "LONG LIFE" to patient.

3.1.2.2 Pharmacological treatment

ICMR guidelines (2005) and many pharmacology books described the different drugs as Pharmacological treatment of diabetes. The pharmacological treatment includes the treatment with drugs and is focused on controlling and lowering of blood glucose level in body. Drugs clinically used for the treatment of diabetes mainly divided in to Oral hypoglycemic drugs and Insulin therapy.

Oral –hypoglycemic drug

Table 3.2: Oral hypoglycemic drugs act by different mechanism to control the condition of hyperglycemia

Oral hypoglycemic drugs	Mechanism of action
1 Sulphonyl urea • Chloropropamide • Tolbutamide • Glibenclamide • Glipizide	• Increases the insulin secretion
2 Non-sulphonyl urea **A Meglitinide analogues** • Repaglinide • Nateglinide **B Biguanides** • Metformin • Phenformin	• Increases the insulin secretion • Decreases the hepatic output of glucose

3 Alpha-glucosidase inhibitors • Acarbose	• Absorption of Glucose by inhibiting the alpha glucosidase enzyme
4 Thiazolidinedione's • Rosiglitazone • Pioglitazone	• Increases the insulin sensitivity in adipose tissues and skeletal muscle.

Insulin

Insulin therapy is important part of diabetes treatment. It is a peptide hormone secreted by beta cells of pancreas. The main work of insulin is to maintain the blood sugar level within the normal range. Disorder of pancreas resulted in insulin deficiency in body.

Insulin production in body:

Alzira Martins and Lopez (2004) have very well talk about the insulin production in body. Insulin secretes from islet of Langerhans in pancreas that contain hormone producing cells. Islet of Langerhans consists of four types of cells: α (alpha), β (beta), δ (delta) and γ (gamma OR PP) cells. The cells constitute 20% of islet while beta cells exist in large amount (70%) in islets. δ cells forms a very least part of islets (3%).Insulin and glucagon produce from beta and alpha cells. Both the hormone plays an important role in carbohydrate metabolism whereas somatostatin and pancreatic polypeptides are released from delta and gamma cells of islet of Langerhans.

Structure of insulin: Insulin is composed of two chains A and B of 51 amino acids and has molecular weight 5908 Da. The two chains of insulin are linked together by disulphide bonds.

Preparations: Insulin can be divided on the basis of sources, pharmacokinetic property and purity.

Source

- Bovine (beef insulin)
- Porcine (pork insulin)
- Human

Pharmacokinetic properties

- Short acting (Bovine, Porcine and Human) aspart, lispro
- Intermediate acting (Bovine, Porcine, Human) e.g NPH
- Long acting (Bovine, Human) e.g glargine

Purity

- Highly purified insulin
- Monocomponent with impurities less than 1 ppm
-

Actions

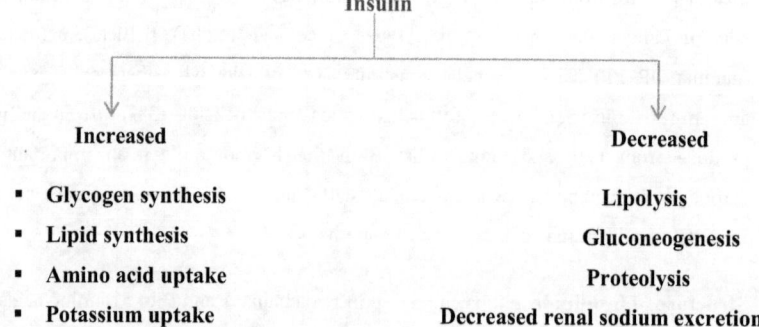

Dimitriadis G (2011) and Clausen T (2008) explained the insulin effect on regulation of translocation of Na+-K+ pumps. Insulin promotes the glycogen synthesis and converts the glucose in to glycogen in the liver cell and reduces the excess level of glucose from the blood. Insulin removes fats from the blood through fat cell and thereby decreases the level of lipid from the blood. Insulin decreases the proteolysis and also causes the reduction in the conversion of stored lipids into blood fatty acids. It stimulates the entry of Na^+, K^+ & PO_4 in to the adipose tissues. It facilitates the transport of glucose across the cell membrane. In this way insulin promotes the different metabolic pathways and maintains the level of glucose with in the normal range.

3.1.2.3 Herbal Treatment for diabetes

From the ancient times plants have been used for food, cloth and as a source of medicines for the treatment of several diseases. Many Plants and plant derived products from ancient times have been used in treating diabetes. Several Phyto-constituents like glycosides, alkaloids, terpenoids, and flavonoids belonging to different classes which serve as main components of plant material and these Phyto-constituents showed their antidiabetic action with different mechanism.

3.1.2.3.1 Phytochemicals for management of Diabetes

WHO has recommended the evaluation of traditional plant treatments for diabetes as they are effective, non-toxic, with less or no side effects and are considered to be excellent aspirants for oral therapy. A scientific validation of several plant species has proved the efficiency of the botanicals in reducing the sugar level. From the reports on their potential effectiveness against diabetes, it is assumed that the phytochemicals have a major role in the management of diabetes, which needs further exploration for the necessary development of drugs and nutraceuticals from natural resources. During the past few years many phytochemicals responsible for anti-diabetic effects have been isolated from the plants. Several Phyto-constituents such as alkaloids, glycosides, flavonoids, saponins, dietary fibers, polysaccharides, glycolipids, peptidoglycans, amino acids and others obtained from various plant sources that have been reported as potent hypoglycemic agents. Here below in table 3.3 listing the potential Phyto-chemicals constituents isolated from plants with their established mechanism of action in the management of diabetes.

Table: 3.3 Phytochemicals with their reported mode of action in managing the diabetes

Plant name	Isolated Phytochemical	Nature of compound	Plant part	Mechanism of action	Reference
*Berberis*L., *Tinosporacardifolia*	Berberine	Alkaloids	Roots and Stem bark	Berberine inhibit the alpha-glucosidase activity and decreases the glucose transport through intestinal epithelium	Singh et al (2003)
Syzygium malaccense	Casuarine 6-O-α-glucoside	Alkaloids	Bark	Casuarine-6-O-α-glucoside inhibit the α-glucosidase activity	Kiyoteru et al (2005)
Catharanthus Roseus	Catharanthine, vindoline and vindolinine	Alkaloids	Leaves and Stem	Lowers the blood glucose level by inhibiting the alpha-glucosidase enzyme	Chattopadhyay et al (1999)
Tribulus terrestris	Harmane and norharmane	Imidazoline alkaloids	Leaves	Isolated alkaloids stimulated the insulin secretion by the activation of imidazole I (3) binding sites in the pancreatic cells. It Stimulate the insulin secretion in glucose dependent manner	Kirtikar et al (1993), Nandkarni A.K (1992)
Syzygium cumini	Jambosine	Alkaloids	Seeds, fruits and bark	It halts the distatic conservation of starch in body.	Murli M.(2011)
Talinum paniculatum	Javaberine A, javaberine A hexaacetate, and javaberine B hexaacetate	Quinolizidine alkaloids	Roots	These isolated alkaloids inhibited the TNF-alpha production by macrophages and fat cells	Catthareeya et al (2013)
*Lepidium sativum*L	Lepidine and semilepidine	Imidazoline alkaloids	Seeds	Lepidine reducing oxidative damage and modulating antioxidant enzymes.	Shukla and Srivastava (2012)
*Lupinus perennis*L	lupanine, 13-α OH-lupanine and 17-oxo-lupanine	Quinolizidine alkaloids	Leaves	Result showed that these alkaloids enhanced glucose-induced insulin release from isolated rat islet cells.	Lopez et al (2004)
Piper	Piperum	Alkaloids	Leaves	Lowers the blood	Tabpoda

umbellatum L.	bellactamA,piperum bellactam B, piperumbellactam C			glucose level by inhibiting the alpha-glucosidase enzyme	et al (2008)
Murrayakoe nigii(L.)	Mahanimbine	Carbazole alkaloid	Leaves	It enhances the insulin release.	Dinesh et al (2010)
Penaresschu lzei	Schulzeines A, B andC	Isoquinoline alkaloids	Leaves	Lowers the blood glucose level by inhibiting the alpha-glucosidase enzyme	Takada et al (2004)
M. alba	1-deoxynojirimycin	Polyhydroxyla tedpiperidine alkaloid	Leaves and bark	It showed antidiabetic activity by inhibiting α-glycosidase inhibitors	Asano et al (2001)
Syzygium cumini	Jamboline	Glycosides	Seeds	It showed hypoglycemic action by inhibiting the conversion of starch into sugar.	Yarnell et al (2009)
Myrcia multiflora DC	Myrciacitrins I and II	Glycosides	Leaves	It showed antidiabetic activity by inhibiting aldose reductase and alpha-glucosidase enzyme.	Matsuda et al (2002)
Ficus bengalensis L	Dimethoxy derivative of perlargonidin 3-O- α - L rhamnoside	Glycosides	Bark	It showed re-generation of β-cells of pancreas and increase the secretion of insulin	Cherian et al (1992)
Polygonatu msp.	PO-1 and PO-2	Steroidal glycosides	Rhizom es	It decreases the absorption of glucose.	Kato et al (1996)
Anemarrhen a asphodeloid es	PseudoprototinosaponinAIII&prototinosaponin AIII	Glycosides	Rhizom es	It showed hypoglycemic effect by their actions on hepatic gluconeogenesis or on glycogenolysis	Toshihiro et al (2001)
Microcospa niculataL.	Vitexin, isovitexin, and isorhamnetin3-O-β-Drutinoside	Flavonoid glycosides	Leaves	It showed antidiabetic effect by inhibiting α-glucosidase enzyme.	Chen .Y.G et al (2013)
Pterocarpus marsupium	epicatechin	Flavonoids	Heart wood	It showed effective insulin mimetic action	Patel et al (2012)
Bergeniacili ata	(-)-3-O galloylepicatechin and (-)-3-Ogalloylcatechin.	Flavonoids	Leaves	It gives the significant anti-diabetic activity and showed inhibitory activities against intestinal α – glucosidase enzyme	Zang et al (2011)
Chamaecost us cuspidatus	Quercetin	Flavonoids	Leaves	It inhibit the plasma cholesterol, triglycerides and increases the hepatic	Hii and Howell et al (1995)

Plant	Compound	Class	Part	Activity	Reference
				glucokinase activity	
Pterocarpus marsupium	Marsupsin, pterosupin and pterostilbene	Flavonoids	Heart wood	It showed potential insulin mimetic activity	Manickam et al (1997)
Psidium guajava L.	Strictinin, isostrictinin and pedunculagin	Flavonoids	Leaves	It showed the hypoglycemic activity by increases the sensitivity of Insulin.	Chauhan et al (2010)
Andrographis paniculata	Andrographolide	Diterpenoid lactone	Leaves	It showed the hypoglycemic activity by increasing plasma beta-endorphin like immunoreactivity (BER) dose	Yu et al (2008)
Zanthoxylum gilletii	3β-Acetoxy-16 β - hydroxybetulinic acid and 3β, 16 β-diacetoxybetulinicacid	Pentacyclic triterpene acetates	Stem bark	These triterpenes showed potent α-glucosidase inhibiting activity	M baze et al (2007)
Bumelia sartorum	Bassic acid	Unsaturated triterpene acid	Root bark	It showed antidiabetic activity by increasing glucose uptake and glycogen synthesis	Naik et al (1991)
Momordica charantia L.	Charantin	Steroidal saponin,	Seeds	It showed antidiabetic activity by stimulating insulin secretion and inhibiting the formation of glucose in blood.	Ng T.B et al (1986)
Lagerstroemia speciosa(L.)	Colosolic acid and maslinic acid	Terpenoids	Leaves	This terpenoids is acting as active glucose transport.	Judy et al (2003)
Gymnema sylvestre	Gymnemic acid IV	Pentacyclic triterpenoid	Leaves	It increases the glucose uptake in muscles, insulin secretion in pancreatic-β-cells.	Sugihara et al (2000)
Coleus forskohlii	Forskolin	Diterpene	leaves	It increases the glucose induced insulin secretion	Wiedenkeller and Sharp et al **(1983)**
Azadirachta indica	β-sitosterol	Steroid	Leaves	It showed hypoglycemic activity by inducing the secretion of insulin	http://nomorediabetes.org/121/better-your-betasitosterol
Curcuma longa	Ferulic acid	4-hydroxy-3-methoxycinnamic acid	Leaves	It showed stimulatory effect in insulin secretion	Nomura et al (2003)
Panax ginseng	Ginseng polypeptides	Polypeptide	Roots	It showed antidiabetic effect by decreasing the	Kimura et al (1981)

				Liver glycogen	
Aralia elata	Elatosides E	Saponin	Root cortex	It showed potent hypoglycemic activity in oral glucose tolerance test in rats.	Yoshikawa et al (1995)
Allium sativum	S-allyl cysteine sulphoxide, (allicin),	Amino acid	Bulb	It showed potential antidiabetic activity equivalent to glibenclamide	Kumari et al (1995)
Swertia japonica	Bellidifolin	Xanthone	Leaves	It increases the glucose uptake activity	Basnet et al (1995)
Salacia reticulata	Kotalanol	Xanthone	Roots and stem	It showed potent alpha glucosidase inhibitory activity	Yoshikawa et al (1995)
Curcuma longa L.	Curcuminoids	Diarylheptanoid	Rhizomes	It is proved to be remarkable alpha glucosidase inhibitor	Du, Z.Y. et al (2006)
Medicago sativa	Manganese chloride	Salt	Leaves	Manganese act as cofactor for ATP phosphorylation of the 3-subunit of the insulin receptor	Luo et al (1998) and Rubenstein et al (1962)

Here In above table only the plants constituents with established mode of actions are listed however there are many more constituents isolated from plants and possess good antidiabetic activity.

Table: 3.4 Some Phyto-constituents with their well-known mode of action

Phyto-constituents	Mode of action
Alkaloids	Inhibit the alpha-glucosidase enzyme and decrease the glucose transport through intestine.
Imidazoline compound	Stimulate the insulin secretion in glucose dependent manner.
Polysaccharides	Increase the serum insulin level
Flavonoids	Suppress the glucose level, reduces the plasma cholesterol.
Dietary fibers	Adsorb the glucose; inhibit the activity of alpha amylase.
Saponins	Stimulates the release of insulin and block the formation of glucose in blood streams.

Ferulic acid	Stimulate insulin secretion

Plants have always been good source of medicines. The ethno botanical survey reports that 800 m plants possess antidiabetic potential. In Indian traditional system of medicine from time of *Charaka*, *Sushruta* plants have been used in diabetes treatment. Most of the experiments studies to examine the antidiabetic activity of plants are carried out on rodents. Patel et al (2011) in their review have collated the different medicinal plants used in treatment of diabetes.

Table 3.5: Summary of antidiabetic plants whose study has already been conducted on STZ induced diabetic rats

Plant name	Family	Part used	Observation (Extract with significant antidiabetic dose)
Afzelia africana	Fabaceae	Stem bark	Aqueous extract of stem bark of plant showed antidiabetic activity at 100 and 200 mg/kg. Best dose is 200 mg/kg.
Allium cepa	Liliaceae	Aerial part	Essential oil (100 mg/kg) gives significant antidiabetic activity.
Amaranthas caudatus	Amaranhacea	Leaves	Methanolic extract (200 and 400 mg/kg b. wt) significantly showed action.
Andrographis lineata	Acanthaceae	Leaves	Methanol and aqueous extracts (400 mg/kg) reduces the blood glucose level.
Annona squamosa	Annonaceae	Leaves	Ethanolic extract (100 mg/kg) produce significant results.
Artocarpus heterophyllus	Moraceae	Leaves	Ethanolic extracts of plants (400 mg/kg) significantly reduces the blood glucose level.
Asystasia gangetica	Acanthaceae	Leaves	Ethanolic extracts (100 and 200 mg/kg) reduces the blood glucose level.

Boerhaavia diffusa	*Nyctaginsceae*	Root	Ethanolic extract at 100 mg and 200 mg-significant action
Berberis vulgaris	*Berberidaceae*	Leaves	Aqueous extracts (62.5 mg and 25.0 mg)and saponins - significant action
Brassica Junceae	*Brassicaceae*	Seeds	Aqueous extract (250 mg,350 mg and 450 mg)
Caesalpinia Bonduc	*Fabaceae*	Seeds	Hydro-methanolic extract showed significant action.
Caesalpinia Digyna	*Caesalpiniaceae*	Leaves	Methanolic extract (250 mg and 500 mg).
Cassia auriculata	*Leguminoseae*	Leaves	Aqueous leaf extracts (400 mg).
Cassia glauca	*Caesalpiniaceae*	Leaves and bark	Aqueous extract (500 mg)
Cassia siamea	*Fabaceae*	Leaves	Methanolic extract(250 mg and 500 mg)
Cinnnamomum zeylanicum	*Lauraceae*	Leaves	Aqueous leaf extracts (30 mg).
Cleome aspera	*Capparaceae*	Whole plant	Methanolic extract (400 mg).
Clitoria ternatea	*Fabaceae*	Whole plant	Aqueous extract (100 mg).
Coccinia indica	*Cucurbitaceae*	Fruits	Ethanolic extract of fruits (200 mg and 400 mg).
Cucumis sativus	*Cucurbitaceae*	Fruits	Ethanolic extract (200 mg and 400 mg)
Dodonaea viscosa	*Sapindaceae*	Whole plants	Water extract and polar fraction of ethanolic extract(400 mg)
Enicostemma littorale	*Gentianaceae*	Leaves	Aqueous extract (1g)
Eucalyptus globules	*Myrtaceae*	Leaves	Alcoholic extract (0.05,0.10,0.20 and 0.40 g/kg p.o)

Hoarrhena antidysenterica	Apocynaceae	Seeds	Methanolic extract (250 mg/kg)
Hypericum Perforatum	Hypericaceae	Whole plants	Ethyl acetate extract (50,100 and 200 mg/kg)
Lawsonia inermis	Lythraceae	Leaves	Ethanolic extract (150,300 and 500mg/kg)
Morus alba	Moraceae	Leaves	Aqueous extract (100,200 and 400 mg)
Nyctanthes arbor-tristis	Oleaceae	Leaves	Ethanol extract (250 and 500 mg)
Olea europaea	Oleaceae	Leaves	Alcohol extract (0.10,0.25 and 0.50 g/kg)
Punica granatum	Lamiaceae	Peels	Hydro-alcoholic extract (400 mg)
Rhus coriaria	Anacardiaceae	Leaves	Ethanolic extract (200 mg)
Rosa canina	Rosaceae	Fruits	Ethanolic extract (250 mg)
Salmalia malabrica	Bombacaceae	Sepals	Hydro-methanolic extract (2:3 v/v)
Stachytarpheta Indica	Verbenaceace	Leaves	Ethanolic extract (300 mg and 600 mg)
Swietenia macrophylla	Meliaceae	Seeds	Methanolic extract (200 and 300 mg)
Syzygium cumini	Myrtaceae	Seeds	Petroleum ether, chloroform, acetone, Methanol (100 mg)
Terminalia bellerica	Combretaceae	Fruits	Hexane, Ethyl acetate and methanol extract (200,300 and 400 mg)
Terminalia superba	Combretaceae	Leaves	Methanol/methylene chloride extract (200,400 mg/kg p.o)
Tinospora cordifolia	Menispermacea	Stem	Hexane, ethyl acetate and methanol extract (250 mg)

Literature search have shown that prominent part of plant which showed antidiabetic activity are leaves. About 44 % percent leaves showed the antidiabetic effect as compare to flowers, bulbs, fruits, roots and seeds.

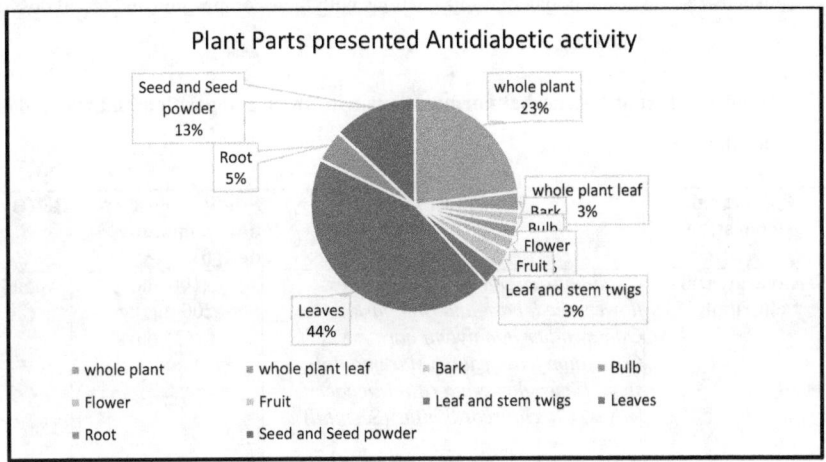

Figure 3.1: Antidiabetic activity distributed in plants parts

3.2 Polyherbal formulations: Literature search on clinical and experimental studies on Antidiabetic polyherbal formulations

Ayurvedic science is the traditional science of India. The belief of Ayurveda is to protect the human being from unnecessary suffering and providing the healthy long life. Ayurvedic science helps to remove the basic cause of the disease with the use of natural elements. It restores the imbalances of body in disease condition and prevents its' re-occurrence. Generally, three classes of medicines i.e. herbal, mineral and animal are derived from Ayurvedic sciences. In these Herbal medicines are gaining popularity worldwide. In Ayurvedic herbal medicines used in two ways either as single herb or as multiple herbs called as "Polyherbalism". It is one of the wonderful concepts given by Ayurveda. The Ayurvedic literature '*Sarangdhar Samhita*' featured the concept of polyherbalism to achieve greater therapeutic efficacy. Subramani et al (2014) cited the different examples in their review to believe that when two herbs combine in particular ratio then result in desire therapeutic effect will be much better as compared to single herbal plant. Till now many polyherbal formulations have been developed, evaluated and used in the management of diabetes. Some of the polyherbal formulations with their composition and tested dose(s) are described below in Table 3.6

Table 3.6: List of Polyherbal Formulations with their composition and tested dose for antidiabetic activity

Polyherbal preparation	Composition	Studied dose with duration(study design)	Reference
Aavaraiyathi churnam	Cassia auriculata (Aavarai) leaves, flower, seed, bark and root bark, Odinawodier (Odhiyam) bark, Coscinium fenestratum(Maramanjal) stem, Ficus glomerata (Atthi) tender leaves, Cocculuscordifolius (Seenthil) stem	100 and 200 mg/kg for 21 days	Anbu N et al (2012)
Cogent db	Azardirachta indica, Curcuma longa, Phyllanthus emblica, Rotula aquatic, Syzigium cumini, Terminalia chebula, Terminalia bellerica, Tribulus terrestris, Trigonella foenum graecum	0.15-0.45g/kg for 40 days	Pari L et al (2004)
Dihar	Syzygium cumini, Momordica charantia, Emblica officinalis, Gymnema sylvestre, Enicostemm, Azadirachta indiaca, Tinosporacordifolia and Curcuma longa	100 and 200 mg for 6 weeks	Patel et al (2009)
Diabet	Curcuma longa, Coscinium fenestratum, Strychnospotatorum, Phyllanthus reticulatus. Tamarindus indica, Tribulusterrestris	500 mg for seven days	Umamaheswariet al (2009)
Diasol	Eugenia jambolana, Foenumgraceum, Terminalia chebula, Quercus, infectoria, Cuminumcyminum, Taraxacumofficinale,	125 and 250 mg for 14 days	Shahul et al (2010)

	Emblica officinalis, Gymnea sylvestre, Phyllanthusnerui and Enicostemmalittorale		
Diakyur	Cassia javanica, Cassiaauriculata, Salacia reticulate, Gymnema sylvestre, Mucunapruriens, Syzygium jambolaum, Terminalia arjuna	1600 mg for 28 days	Joshi et al (2007)
Diasulin	Cassia auriculata, Coccinia indica, Curcuma longa, Emblica officinalis, Gymnema sylvestre, Momordica charantia, Scopariadulcis, Syzygium cumini, Tinospora cordifolia, Trigonella foenum graecum	200 mg for 30 days	Pari et al (2004)
Diabecon	Gymnema sylvestre, Pterocarpus marsupium, Glycyrrhiza glabra, Casearia esculenta, Syzygium cumini, Asparagus racemosus, Boerhavia diffusa, Sphaeranthus indicus, Tinospora cordifolia, Swertia chirata, Tribulus terrestris, Phyllanthus amarus, Gmelinaarborea, Gossypium herbaceum, Berberis aristata, Aloe vera, Triphala, Commiphora wightii, shilajeet, Momordica charantia, Piper nigrum, Ocimum sanctum, Abutilon indicum, Curcuma longa, Rumexmaritimus	2 tablets twice a day for 12 weeks	Yajnik et al (1993)
Dia-Care	Eugenia jambolona, Tinospora cordifolia, Gymnema sylvestre, Cressacretica, Csekriaesculenta, Curcuma longa, Trigonella fonumgraecum, Terminaliachebula, Holarrhen aantidysenterica, Pterocarpus marsupium, Mineral pitch, Tribulusterrestris, Withania somnifera, Nordotachym jatamansi, Bocopa monniera.	250 and 500 mg for 15 days	Reddy et al (2012)
Diabeta	Gymnema sylvestre, Vincarosea(Periwinkle), Curcuma longa	2.5 mg and 5 mg	Modak et al (2012)

	(Turmeric), *Azadirachta indica* (Neem), *Pterocarpus marsupium* (Kino Tree), *Momordica chara*ntia (Bitter Gourd), *Syzygium cumini*(Black Plum), *Acacia arabica*(BlackBabhul), *Tinospora cordifolia*, *Zingiber officinale*(Ginger)		
ESF/AY/500	*Aervalanata, Aegle marmelos, Ficus benghalensis, Catharanthus roseus, Bambus aarundinaceae, Salacia reticulate and Szygium cumini* and *'Eruca sativa'*	100 mg and 500 mg for 21 days	Sajeeth et al (2002)
5EPHF	*Aegelmarmelos*(root), *Aloe vera*(leave), *Elaeodendronglaucum*(leave), *Murrayakoenigii*(root), *Pongamiapinnata*(stem bark)	50 – 200 mg for 21 days	Lanjhiyana et al (2011)
Glycoherb	Arogyavardhini, *Azadirachta indica*, Bang bhasma, *Curcuma longa*, Chanraprabha,Devdar, *Gymnema sylvestre*, Harde, *Holarrhena antidysenterica*, Mahamejva,*Momordica charantia, Phyllanthus emblica, Psidium guajava, Sauropusandrogynus,Swertia chirata, Tribulus terrestris Trigonella foenum-graecum*	200,400 and 600 mg for 28 days	Thakkar and Patel (2010)
Glucolevel	*Atriplexhalimus*(leave), *Juglansregia*(leave), *Olea europea*(leave), *Urticadioica*(leave)	1 tablet 3 times a day for 4 weeks	Said O et al (2008)
HAL(14)	*Withaniasomnifera*(root) *Momordica charantia* (fruit), *Trigonella foenum-graecum*(seed)	250-1000 mg/kg for 21 days	Gauttam and Kalia(2013)
Hyponidd	*Cassia auriculata, Curcuma longa, Emblica officinalis, Enicostemmalittorale, Eugenia jambolana, Gymnema sylvestre, Melia Azadirachta, Momordica charantia, Pterocarpus marsupium, TinosporaCordifolia*	100-200 mg for 45 days	Babu et al (2004)

Karmin Plus	Momordica charantia, Azadirachta indica, Picrorrhizakurroa, Ocimum sanctum and Zinziberofficinale	200 or 400 mg for 11days	Bangar et al (2009)
MAC-ST/001	Azadirachta indica (seed), Caesalpiniabonducella(seed), Momordica charantia (fruit), Syzygium cumini (seed), Trigonella foenum-graecum(seed)	100-400 mg for 20 days	Yadav et al (2013)
Niddwin	Tinosporacordifolia, Gymnema sylvestre, Terminalia tomentosa, Asphaltum, Tribulusterrestris, Emblica officinalis, Mucunapruriens, Sidacordifolia, Withania somnifera, Terminalia belerica, Terminalia chebula, Momordica charantia	50 and 100 mg for 10 days	Shruthi et al (2014)
Okchun-San	Coixlachryma-jobi(or Oryza sativa),Glycyrrhiza auralensis, Pueraria,thunbergiana, Rehmanniaglutinosa, Schizandrachinensis, Trichosantheskirilowii	200 mg for 12 days	Chang MS et al (2006)
Okudiabet	Stachytarphetaangustifolia, Alstoniacongensis bark and Xylopiaacthiopicafruits	250 and 500 mg for 31 days	Ogbonnia et al (2011)
SR10(20)	Radix Astragali(root), Radix Codonopsis (root), Cortex Lycii(root)	927 mg/kg for 4 weeks	Chan JY et al (2009)
Ziabeen	Aloe barbadensis, Azadirachta indica, Eugenia jambolana, Gymnema sylvestre, Momordica charantia, Holarrhena antidysenterica, Piper nigrum, Swertia chirata,	2-4 g/kg for 30 days	Akhtar et al (2011)

3.3 PLANT PROFILE

Plants used in developing the polyherbal formulations for present study are as follows:

1. *Morus alba* (leaves)
2. *Annona squamosa* (leaves)
3. *Nelumbo nucifera* (leaves)
4. *Psidium guajava (leaves)*
5. *Coccinia indica (leaves)*
6. *Gymnea sylvestre (leaves)*
7. *Pterocarpus marsupium (heartwood)*
8. *Syzium cumini (seeds)*
9. *Momordica charantia (fruits)*
10. *Piper longum (fruits)*

Chapter 3 — Literature Review

Title: *Morus alba*   **Family:** *Moraceace*

Common Name: White Mulberry, Silkworm mulberry, murier (F), morera (Sp.), tut (Urdu, Farsi, Hindi)

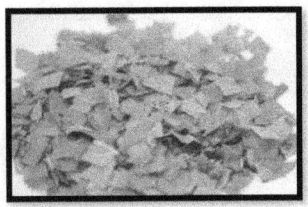

Distribution: Cultivated nationwide, found in old fields, along road sides, forest edges.

Phytochemical Review: *Morus alba* rich in number of phyto-chemicals like Phenolic compound, Alkaloids, Glycosides and Flavonoids.

Table 3.7: Phytochemical Review on Isolated Phyto-constituents from *Morus alba*

Year	Part Used	Isolated Phytoconstituents	Source
2001	Leaves	Two novel prenylflavanes and a glycoside along with six known compounds, isoquercitrin, astragalin, scopolin, skimming, roseoside II and benzyl D-glucopyranoside	Doi k etal
2006	Leaves	rutin, isoquercitrin, astragalin and quercetin-3-(6-malonyl) glucoside among which quercetin - 3-(6-malonyl) glucoside is most abundant in dried mulberry leaf extract.	Katsube et al.
2008	Leaves	Flavonoids	Fu An Wu et al
2009	Root bark	Phenolics i.e Moracin M(100 mg/kg), Steppogenin-4'-O-beta-D-glucosiade(50 mg/kg), Mullberroside A(100 mg/kg)	Zhang M et al
2010	Leaves and fruits	phenolic content and sugar content	Memon et al
2010	Root Bark	Albanol A (was evaluated for the cytotoxic and apoptosis-inducing activities in human leukemia (HL60) cells)	Kikuchi et al
2011	Leaves	A new bioactive compound 3',5'- dihydroxy-6-methoxy-7-prenyl-2-arylbenzofuran	Yang et al
2012	Leaves	Quercetin 3-O-β-glucopyranoside-7-O-α-rhamnopyranoside, kaempferol-7-O-glucoside and	Thabti et al

| | | quercetin-3-O-rhamnopyranoside-7-Oglucopyranoside. | |

Pharmacological Review:

Plant is rich in number of biological activities like antimicrobial, antistress, antidiabetic, hepatoprotective, antihyperlipidemic, anti-oxidant, neuroprotective:

Table 3.8: Pharmacological Activities of *Morus alba*

Year	Plant part	Pharmacological activity	Observation/chemical constituents responsible for activity	Source
1980, 2003	Bark	Anti–microbial activity.	Bioactive molecules from mulberry bark, sanggenon B and D, Morusin and kuwanon C showed antimicrobial activity.	Park et al, Nomura et al
1995	Root bark	Anti-HIV Activity	Flavonoids like mulberrofuran D, mulberrofuran G, mulberrofuran K., morusin, and kwanon G, kwanon H and their derivative presents only morusin, morusin 4′-glucoside and kuwanon H showed activity against HIV.	Shi-De et al
1958, 2004	Leaves and Root Bark	Anti hyperglycemic Activity	Trigonelline and high fiber contents in mulberry leaves.A polyhydroxylatedpiperidine alkaloid, 1-deoxynojirimycin (DNJ) isolated from leaves and root bark of *M. alba* have significant α-glycosidase inhibitors activity.	Watanabe et al Syvacy and Sokmen, et al
2004	Roots	Anti-cancer activity	Prenylated flavanone, 7, 2', 4', 6'-tetrahydoroxy geranylflavanone separated from ethyl acetate extracts of *M.alba* root showed cytotoxic activity against hepatoma cells in rat	Kofujita et al
2008, 2002	Leaves	Antioxidant Activity	quercetin 3-(6-malonylglucoside) is most significant for antioxidant potential of mulberry plant, oxyresveratrol and 5,7-dihydroxycoumarin 7-methyl ether	Butt et al, Oh et al.

| | | | which scavenge superoxide and also have antioxidant potential. | |

Title: *Annona squamosa* **Family:** *Annonacea*

Common name: Sugar apple

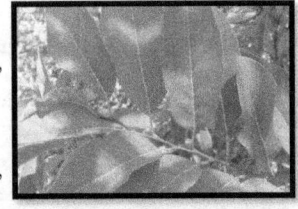

Distribution: Native to tropical Americas and West-Indes, widely cultivated in Indonesia, Thailand, India.

Phytochemical Review: The plant is rich in glycoside, alkaloids, saponins, flavonoids, tannins, carbohydrates, proteins, phenolic compounds, phytosterols, and amino acids. The numbers of chemical constituents have been isolated from *Annona squamosa* like anonaine, aporphine, coryeline, isocorydine, norcorydine, glaucine from leaves, stem and roots of plant.

Table 3.9: Phytochemical Review on Isolated Phyto-constituents from *Annona squamosa*

Year	Part Used	Isolated Phytochemical	Source
1996	Fruits	Yielded 12 known kaurane derivatives and two new kauranediterpenoids, which have been named annosquamosin A (16 beta-hydroxy-17-acetoxy-ent-kauran-19-al) and annosquamosin B (19-nor-ent-kaurane-4 alpha, 16 beta,-17-triol).	Wu YCet al
2001	Fruit	Bullatacin, isolated from the fruit of Annona family	ChihHw et al
2008	Leaves	4-(2-nitro-ethyl 1)-1-6-((6-o-β-Dxylopyranosyl-β-D-glucopyranosyl) oxy)benzene,Anonaine, Benzyltetrahydroisoquinoline, Borneol, Camphene, Camphor, car-3-ene, Carvone, β-Caryphyllene, Eugenol, Farnesol, Geraniol, 16-Hetriacontanone, Hexacontanol, Higemamine,Isocorydine, Limonine, Linalool acetate,	Patel et al
2011	Roots	It contain essential oil (0.15%); β caryophyllene, α pinene, α-humulene, α-gurjunene. Chloroform extract of the plant contains an active constituent	Pandey et al

Year	Plant part	Pharmacological activity	Observation	Source
2012	Leaves	Annotemoyin Isolated the two chemical constituents from the methanolic extract of *Annona Squamosa* which was characterized as characterized as Trim ethyl Ellagic acid and 11, 12 dimethoxy, 2-rhamnosyl, 4-ol, 5-keto flavone.		Gupta et al

Pharmacological Review

Table 3.10: Pharmacological Activities of *Annona squamosa*

Year	Plant part	Pharmacological activity	Observation	Source
2008	Leaves	Antibacterial Activity	Linalool, Borneol, Eugenol, Farnesol, and Geraniol showed antibacterial activity	Patel et al
2008	Leaves	Anti-diabetic Activity	quercetin-3-O-glucoside isolated from leaf showed antidiabetic activity	Sunanda Panda et al
2008	Leaves	Antioxidant Activity	quercetin-3-O-glucoside isolated from leaf showed antioxidant activity	Sunanda Panda et al
2009	Leaves	Hepatoprotective	Ethanolic extract of leaves showed hepatoprotective activity.	Raj et al
2012	Seeds	Antitumor Activity	Annonaceousacetogenin compounds in the extract. 12, 15-cis-squamostatin-A and bullatacin. inhibited the growth of H(22) tumor cells in mice	Chen Y et al
2013	Fruit peel	Anti-hyperlipidemic Activity	alcoholic extract of fruit peel *Annona squamosa* showed antihyperlipidemic activity	Sharma et al

Title: *Nelumbo nucifera*   **Family:** *Nelumbonaceae*

Common names: Indian lotus, sacred lotus, bean of India.

Distribution: *Nelumbo nucifera* is native to tropical Asia and Queensland Australia, wetlands, found in ponds, lakes

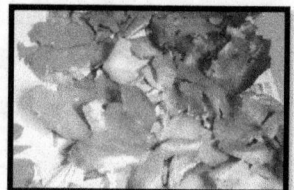

and pools.

Phytochemical Review: *Nelumbo nucifera*is commonly called as lotus. A number of phytochemical constituents' alkaloids, flavonoids, glycosides, fatty acids have been reported from the plant.

Table 3.11: Phyto-chemical Review on Isolated Phytoconstituents from *Nelumbo nucifera*

Year	Part Used	Isolated Phyto-constituents	Source
2004	Leaves	(+)-1(R)-Coclaurine (1) and (−)-1(S)-norcoclaurine, together with quercetin 3-O-β-D-glucuronide were isolated from the leaves of *Nelumbo nucifera* (Nymphaceae), and identified as anti-HIV principles.	YoshikiKashiwada et al
2008	Leaves	Isoquercitrin, hyperoside and astragalin.	Shengguo Deng et al
2009	Leaves	isolation of five nor sesquiterpenes, four flavonoids, two triterpenes and one alkaloid from methanolic extract	Kang Ro Lee et al
2011	Embryos of the seeds	Bisbenzylisoquinoline alkaloids: nelumboferine and nelumborines A and B were isolated along with four known compounds, neferine, liensinine, isoliensinine and anisic acid.	Itoh A et al
2013	Leaves	Isolation of 13 megastigmanes, including a new megastigmane, nelumnucifoside A, and a new eudesmane sesquiterpene, nelumnucifoside B, eight alkaloids and 11 flavonoids.	Ahn JHet al
2013	Leaves	nuciferine (0.34-0.63%), (-)-armepavine (0.13-0.20%), and (+)-isoliensinine (0.06-0.19%	Do TC et al

Pharmacological Review

Table 3.12: Pharmacological Activities of *Nelumbo nucifera*

Year	Plant Part	Pharmacological activity	Observation	Source
1995	Rhizomes	Anti-diarrheal activity	Methanolic extract of rhizomes of Nelumbo nucifera showed significant effect against castor oil induced diarrhea	Mukherjee P K et al
1996	Rhizomes	Antipyretics	Methanolic extract of rhizomes of *Nelumbo nucifera* showed antipyretic activity	Mukherjee PK, et al
1997	Rhizomes	Anti-inflammatory effects	Betulinic acid, a steroidal triterpenoid isolated from rhizomes of *Nelumbo nucifera* have anti-inflammatory activity. This activity was compared with phenylbutazone and dexamethasone.	Mukherjee PK, et al
2005	Leaves	Anti-infective effects	(+)-1(R)-Coclaurine and (-)-1(S)-norcoclaurine, together with quercetin 3-O-beta-D-glucuronide, were isolated from the leaves of *Nelumbo nucifera* (Nymphaceae), and identified as anti-HIV principles.	Kashiwada Y et al
2006	Seeds	Antioxidant effects	Hydro-alcoholic extract of seeds of *Nelumbo nucifera* showed antioxidant activity.	Rai S et al
2009	Seeds embryo	Antidiabetic effects	Neferine showed antidiabetic effect isolated from green seed embryo of *Nelumbo nucifera* Gaertn has an anti-obesity activity. Ethanolic extract of leaves also showed antihyperglycemic activity.	Pan Y et al
2010	Flowers	Antiplatelet activity	Hydro-ethanolic extract of flowers showed dose dependent antiplatelet activity	Durairaj et al

Chapter 3 — Literature Review

Title: *Psidium guajava* **Family:** *Myrtaceae*

Common names: Yellow guava, Lemon guava.

Distribution: It is a native of Central America, South America, Caribbean and widely cultivated in India.

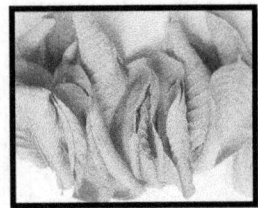

Phytochemical Review: It contains tannins, triterpenes, flavonoid: quercetin, pentacyclictriterpenoid: guajanoic acid, saponins, carotenoids, lectins, leucocyanidin, ellagic acid, amritoside, beta-sitosterol, uvaol, oleanolic acid and ursolic acid. (Kamath et al)

Table 3.13: Phytochemical Review on Isolated Phyto-constituents from *Psidium guajava*

Year	Part Used	Phytochemical constituents	Source
2004	Leaves	One new pentacyclic triterpenoid guajanoic acid and four known compounds beta-sitostero, uvaol, oleanolic acid, and ursolic acid have been isolated from the leaves of *Psidiumguajava*.	Begum S et al
2009	Leaves	Leaves reported to contain Ursolic acid, 2-alpha-hydroxyursolic acid, 2-alpha-hydroxyoleanolic acid, morin-3-O-alpha-L-arabopyranoside, quercetin, hyperin, myricetin-3-O-beta-D-glucosid, quercetin-3-O-beta-D glucuronopyranoside, 1-O-galloyl-beta-D-glucose.	Fu H et al
2010	Leaves	Two triterpenoids betulinic acid and lupeol from the leaf extract of *Psidium guajava* and their potential antimicrobial and phytotoxic activities studied.	P Ghosh
2010	Leaves	Five flavonoidal compounds were isolated which are quercetin, quercetin-3-O-α-L-arabinofuranoside, quercetin-3-O-β-D-arabinopyranoside, quercetin-3-O-β-D-glucoside and quercetin-3-O-β-D-galactoside. Quercetin-3-O-b-D-arabinopyranoside was isolated for the first time from the leaves.	Am.Metwally et al
2014	Fruit	Carbonyls and esters such as 3-hydroxy-2-butanone, 2-heptanone, benzaldehyde, ethyl	Fang Wang et al

		hexanoate, (Z)-3-hexenyl acetate, hexyl butanoate and ethyl octanoate were found only in the fruit.	
2014	Seeds	Macronutrients and micronutrients, with a high content of total dietary fiber (63.94 g/100g), protein (11.19 g/100g), iron (13.8 mg/100g), zinc (3.31 mg/100g), and reduced calorie content (182 kcal/100g). Their lipid profile showed a predominance of unsaturated fatty acids (87.06%), especially linoleic acid (n6) and oleic acid (n9). The powder contained ascorbic acid (87.44 mg/100g), total carotenoids (1.25 mg/100 g) and insoluble dietary fiber (63.55 g/100g).	Ana Maria AthaydeUchôa-thomazet al

Pharmacological Review

Table 3.14: Pharmacological Activities of *Psidium guajava*

Year	Plant Part	Pharmacological activity	Observation	Source
1994	Leaves	Anti-mutagenic activity	(+)-gallocatechin was isolated as a bio-antimutagenic compound found active against UV-induced mutation in Escherichia coli.	T.Matsuo et al
2001	Fruits	Anti-diarrhoeal	Lectin in guava binds to E. coli (a common diarrhea-causing organism) and prevents its adhesion to intestinal wall.	Rodriguez et al
2006	Leaves	Antimicrobial activity	The active flavonoid compound - quercetin-3-O-alpha-l-arabinopyranoside (guaijaverin) - extracted from leaves has high potential antiplaque activity by inhibiting the growth of *Streptococcus mutans*	Prabu GR et al
2006	Leaves	Hepatoprotective activity	Aqueous extract of plant showed hepatoprotective activity against liver injury induced by CCl_4,Paracetamol	Roy et al
2012	Leaves	Anti-diabetic activity	The methanolic extract showed a significant inhibitory effect on glucose diffusion in vitro thus validating the traditional claim of the plant.	Basha et al

| 2014 | Leaves | Anti-inflammatory activity | Leaf extract significantly reduced the lipopolysaccharides induced prostaglandin in dose dependent manner | Jang.M.et al |

Title: *Coccinia indica*

Common names: baby watermelon, little gourd, Kundru

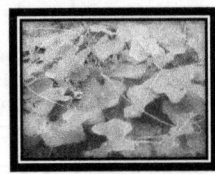

Distribution: All species occur in sub-Saharan Africa, from semi-arid savannas to rain forests, rarely also mountain forests. The species adapted to these different habitats one to several times independently.

Table 3.15: Phytochemical Review on Isolated Phytoconstituents from *Coccinia indica*

Year	Part Used	Isolated Phytoconstituents	Source
1987	Fruits	Taraxerone, taraxerol, and (24R)-24-ethylcholest-5-en-3β-ol glucoside.	Kundu et al
1990	Whole plant	Aspartic acid, Glutamic Acid, Asparagine, Tyrosine, Histidine, Phenylalanine, Threonine Valine Arginine	Rahman et al
1996, 2001	Roots	Coccinio SIDE-K-saponin isolated from butanol extract, Ombuin 3-O-arabinofuranoside	Vaishnav et al
2014	leaves	Alkaloids-Polyhydroxy and phenanthrene alkaloids	Jambulingam

Pharmacological Review

Table 3.16: Pharmacological activities of *Coccinia indica*

Year	Plant part	Pharmacological activity	Observation	Source

1958	Fruit	Anti-tuberculosis activity	Extract of fruit showed reduction in Tubercular bacteria	Mukherji et al
2003	Leaves	Anti-diabetic activity	Ethanolic extract of leaves showed significant reduction in blood glucose level of STZ induced diabetic rats.	Pari et al
2003	Fruits	Hepatoprotective activity	Ethanolic extract of fruits protect the CCl_4 induced liver injury in rats	Rao et al
2009	Leaves	Ant-inflammatory activity	Aqueous extract of leaves showed significant effect in carrageenan-induced paw edema method	Niazi et al
2009	Leaves	Antipyretic & analgesic activity	Aqueous extract of fresh leaves showed significant reduction in hyperpyrexia in rats	Niazi et al
2010	Leaves	Antibacterial activity	Ethanol and aqueous extract significantly inhibit the skin and gastrointestinal infection	Hussain et al

Title: *Gymnema sylvestre*   **Family:** *Asclepiadaceae*

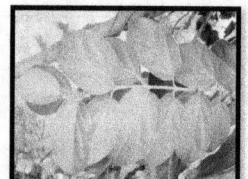

Common names: Gymnema, cow plant, Australian cow plant, gurmari, gurmarbooti, meshasringa, bhetki cha pala.

Distribution: Native to the tropical forests of central and southern India and in scrub jungles.

Phytochemical Review

Table 3.17: Phytochemical Review on Isolated Phytoconstituents from *Gymnema sylvestre*

Year	Part Used	Isolated Phytoconstituents	Source
1971, 1992	Leaves	Saponins such as gymnemic acid deacyl gymnemic acid, gymnemagenin and 23-hydroxylnogispinogenin &gymnestrogenin.	Sinsheimer et al & Yoshikawa et al
1981	Leaves	The individual gymnemic acids (saponins) includegymnemic acids I-VI, gymnemosides A-F and Gymnema saponins.	Chakravarthi et al

1991	Leaves	Gurmarin, an important 35 amino-acid peptide	Ishima et al
2004	Aerial	Gypenoside	Norberg et al
2008	Stem	Isolated the eight compounds from n-butanol extract and identified as Conduritol, 1-Quercitol, Potassium nitrate, Stigmasterol. Chemical compounds1-Heptadecanol, Stigmasterol glucoside, Octadecanol, Lupeol cinnamon are firstly obtained from this plant.	Zhen HS et al

Pharmacological Review

Table 3.18: Pharmacological activities of *Gymnema sylvestre*

Year	Plant part	Pharmacological activity	Observation	Source
2000	Leaves	Anti-diabetic Activity	Saponins fraction and five triterpene glycosides (gymnemic acids and gymnemasaponin) obtained from the methanol extract of leaves of *Gymnema sylvestre*	Sugihara Y et al
2008	Leaves	Anti-Inflammatory Activity	Aqueous extract of leaves reported to contain anti-inflammatory activity	Malik et al
2009	Leaves	Anti-cancer activity	Isolated saponins gymnemagenol showed cytotoxic positive activity against HeLa cells.	Venkatesan et al
2013	Leaves	Anti-microbial Activity	Phytochemical screening resulted in presence of alkaloids, steroids, saponins, tannins from chloroform; hexane and methanol extract and also showed positive effect against gram positive and gram-negative organisms.	Naidu et al
2013	Leaves	Free Radical Scavenging Activity	Give the positive in-vitro antioxidant potential using DPPH	Ahirwal et al
2013	Leaves	Anti-obesity Activity	Water soluble fraction of plant serum lipids, insulin, glucose, apolipoprotein B and LDL	Kumar et al

| | | | levels | |

Title: *Pterocarpus marsupium* **Family:** *Fabaceae*

Common names: Vijayasar or the Indian Kino Tree

Distribution: India, Srilanka, Nepal and WesternGhats in Karnatka-Kerla region.

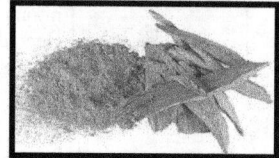

Phytochemical Review

Table 3.19: Phytochemical Review on Isolated Phyto-constituents from *Pterocarpus marsupium*

Year	Part Used	Isolated Phytochemical	Source
1985	Bark	(-)-Epicatechin: flavonoid	Chakravarthy et al
1989	Flower	Aurone glycosides: 4,6,4'-trihydroxyaurone 6-*O*-rhamnopyranoside and 4,6,4'-trihydroxy-7-methylaurone 4-*O*-rhamnopyranoside	Mohan et al
2000	Heartwood	An isoaurone C-glucoside	Handa et al
2000	Heartwood	C glucoside, 1-(2', 6'-dihydroxyphenyl)-β-D-glucopyranoside	Suri et al
2004	Heartwood	Five new flavonoid C-glucosides, 6-hydroxy-2-(4-hydroxybenzyl)-benzofuran-7-C-beta-d-glucopyranoside,3-(alpha-methoxy-4-hydroxybenzylidene)-6-hydroxybenzo-2(3H)-furanone-7-C-beta-d-glucopyranoside,2-hydroxy-2-p-hydroxybenzyl-3(2H)-6-hydroxybenzofuranone-7-C-beta-d-glucopyranoside,8-(C-beta-d-glucopyranosyl)-7,3',4'-trihydroxyflavone and 1,2-bis(2,4-dihydroxy,3-C-glucopyranosyl)-ethanedione and two known compounds C-beta-d-glucopyranosyl-2,6-dihydroxyl benzene and sesquiterpene from aqueous extract.	Maurya et al

Chapter 3

Pharmacology Review

Table 3.20: Pharmacological activities of *Pterocarpus marsupium*

Year	Plant part	Pharmacological activity	Observation	Source
1985	Bark	CNS activity	(-)-Epicatechin: flavonoid showed positive chronotropic and inotropic effects on frog hearts.	Chakravarthy et al
2004	Bark	*Anti-cataract activity*	Aqueous extract of bark decreases the opacity index.	Vats et al
2004	Stem Bark	*Hepatoprotective activity*	Toxic effect of CCl_4 was controlled by methanolic extract if plant by restoring the bilirubin and other liver parameters.	Krishna et al
2005	Bark	*COX-2 Inhibition*	Petro stilbene from bark significantly reduces the prostaglandin synthesis.	Hougee et al
2007	Heartwood	Cardio tonic activity	5,7,2-4 tetrahydroxyisoflavone-6,6-glucoside from aqueous extract significantly increases in height of force of contraction	Mohire et al
2011	Heartwood	*Antidiabetic/ Anti-hyperglycemic /Anti-oxidant activity*	Ethanolic extract of heartwood reduce the blood glucose level, reduce the lipid level and antioxidant enzymes.	Mohan et al

Title: *Syzygium cumini*   **Family:** *Myrtaceae*

Common names: Jamunjambul, jambolan, jamblang

Distribution: Nepal, Pakistan, India, Sri-lanka, Malaysia

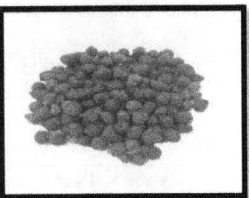

Phytochemical Review

Table 3.21: Phytochemical Review on Isolated Phytoconstituents from *Syzygium cumini*

Year	Part Used	Isolated Phytochemical	Source
1975	Bark, Seeds	Gallic acid, ellagic acid, corilagin and related ellagitannins, 3,6–hexahydroxydiphenoyl-glucose and its isomer, 4,6–hexahydroxydiphenoyl glucose, 1–galloyl glucose, 3–galloyl glucose and Quercetin have been isolated from alcoholic extract of Jambul seeds. Acetone extract of the bark and seeds contain partially methylated derivatives of ellagic acid i.e. 3,3'-di–O–methyl ellagic acid and 3,3', 4–tri–O–methyl ellagic acid.	Bhatia et al
2007	Leaves	Phenolic content	LucileneAzevedo Lima
2012	Leaves	Oil constitutes were α-pinene (17.53%), α-terpineol (16.67 %) and alloocimene (13.55%) in S. cumini, trans-caryophyllene (15.57%) and cedrol (21.29%), Δ3-carene (17.85%) and α-pinene (6.9%) tested against bacteria.	Elansary et al
2012	Leaves	Lupeol, 12-oleanen-3-ol-3ß-acetate, Stigmasterol, ß-sitosterol were identified from n-hexane fraction of plant extract	Md. RashedulAlam
2012	Leaves	7-hydroxycalamenene, methyl-β-orsellinate, β-sitosterol and oleanolic acid from methanolic extract	Rashid et al
2013	Bark, Seed, Leaves	Malieic acid, oxalic acid, gallic acid, tannins, cynidin glycoside, oleanolic acid, flavonoids, essential oils, betulinic acid, friedelin have been identified for antioxidant activity	Ramya et al

Pharmacological Review

Table 3.22: Pharmacological activities of *Syzygium cumini*

Year	Plant Part	Pharmacological activity	Observation	Source
2001	Bark	**Anti-inflammatory**	Ethanolic extract showed anti-inflammatory activity	Muruganandan et al

Year	Part	Activity	Description	Reference
2007	Seed	**CNS activity**	Ethyl acetate and methanol extract of seeds tested in rota rod and actophotometer.	Kumar et al
2007	Skeels	**Anti-allergic activity**	Inhibition of eosinophil accumulation in the allergic pleurisy model is probably due to an impairment of CCL11/eotaxin and IL-5 production.	Brito et al
2012	Seed	**Anti-diabetic activity**	seed extract contain apigenin 7-O-glucoside and leaf extract give Dihydro-3,3',4',5,7 – pentahydroxyflavone glycoside which is identified as α-glucosidase inhibitors	Alagesan et al
2012	Leaves	**Anti-bacterial activity**	Oil constitutes were α-pinene (17.53%), α-terpineol (16.67 %) and alloocimene (13.55%) in S. cumini, trans-caryophyllene (15.57%) and cedrol (21.29%), Δ3-carene (17.85%) and α-pinene (6.9%) tested against bacteria.	Elansary et al
2013	Ariel part	**Antioxidant activity**	malieic acid, oxalic acid, gallic acid, tannins, cynidin glycoside, oleanolic acid, flavonoids, essential oils, betulinic acid, friedelin have been identified for antioxidant activity	Ramya et al

Title: *Momordica charantia*　　**Family:** *Cucurbitaceae*

Common names: Bitter gourd, bitter melon bitter squash or balsam-pea.

Distribution: Asia, Africa, Caribbean, widely distributed all over in India.

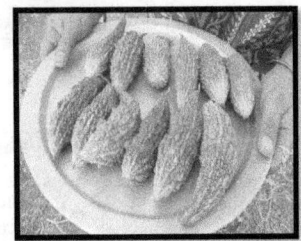

Phytochemical Review

Table 3.23: Phytochemical Review on Isolated Phyto-constituents from *Momordica charantia*

Year	Part Used	Isolated Phytochemical	Source
2002	Leaves, Fruits and Seeds	Different phytochemicals alkaloids, glycosides(charantin),polypeptide-P, Oils from the seeds(linoleic, stearic and oleic acids),glycoproteins isolated from plant and analyzed for hypoglycemic activity	Taylor et al
2004	Seeds	A glycol alkaloid: Vicine showed hypoglycemic action	Haixia et al
2007	Fruit	Charantin, a steroidal saponin having insulin-like properties and momordicin, an alkaloid provide bitterness	Pitipanponga et al
2008	Seeds	*trans*-nerolidol, apiole, *cis*-dihydrocarveol and germacrene D	Braca et al
2009	Fruits	Eight compounds isolated: momordicolide ((10E)-3-hydroxyl-dodeca-10-en-9-olide, monordicophenoide A (4-hydroxyl-benzoic acid 4-O-beta-D-apiofuranosyl -O-beta-D-glucopyranoside, 2), dihydrophaseic acid 3-O-beta-D-glucopyranoside, 6,9-dihydroxy-megastigman-4,7-dien-3-one (blumenol), guanosine, adenosine, uracil and cytosine.	Li QY et al
2008	Leaves	Momordicin 1 chemical structure was characterized as momordicin1 3, 7, 23,-Trihydroxycucurbitan-5,24-dien-19-al	Puspawati et al
2013	Seeds	4a-phorbol-12, 13-didecanoate, Hexane, Ethyl acetate and ethanol extract showed the presence of flavonoids, glycosides, sterols, fat and oil. Hexane and ethyl acetate contain only Anthraquinone. Alkaloids are present in both hexane and ethanol extract.	Oragwa et al

Pharmacological Review

Table 3.24: Pharmacological activities of *Momordica charantia*

Year	Plant Part	Pharmacological activity	Observation	Source
1983	Fruit	Anti-cancer activity	Extract inhibited the formation of tumor cells in mice	Jilka et al

1988	Seeds	Abortifacient activity	Abortifacient proteins trichosanthin, alpha-momorcharin and beta-momorcharin inhibit cell-free protein synthesis in pregnant mice	Yeung et al
2009	Fruit	Anti-ulcer activity	Methanolic extract of fruits showed significant antiulcer activity in acetic acid induced gastric ulcer in rats	Samsul et al
2011	Fruit	Antidiabetic activity	Saponins: Momordicine II and 3-hydroxycucurbita-5, 24-dien-19-al-7, 23- di-O-β-glucopyranoside .These compounds showed significant insulin releasing activity in MIN6 β-cells	Keller et al
2011	Fruit	Antibacterial activity	Ethyl acetate and methanolic fraction showed effective zone of inhibition against E.coli	Costa et al
2011	Seeds, Fruits and Leaves	Anti-HIV activity	Proteins like MAP30 and alpha and beta momocharin obtained from *Momordica charantia* were found to be an effective anti HIV agents	Rashmi et al
2012	Fruit	Analgesic and anti-inflammatory	Oral administration of ethanolic extract of fruits showed analgesic activity in acetic acid induced writhing and carrageenan induced paw edema in rats.	M.Ullah et al
2013	Fruits	Antioxidant activity	Aqueous extract of fruits showed antioxidant effect	Hamissou et al
2014	Fruit	Anti-malarial activity	Chloroform extract of fruit coat of *Momordica charantia* showed good anti-plasmodium activity	Yousif et al
2014	Fruit	Immunomodulatory activity	Polysaccharide of M. charantia (MCP) from the fruits of plants control levels in cyclophosphamide (Cy)-induced immunosuppressed mice	Deng et al

Title: *Piper longum*   **Family:** *Piperaceae*

Common names: Long pepper, Pippali, Pippali

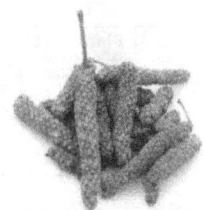

Distribution: Widely distributed all over India, Sri Lanka, Middle Eastern countries and the Americas.

Phytochemical Review

Table 3.25: Phyto-chemical Review on Isolated Phyto-constituents from *Piper longum*

Year	Part Used	Isolated Phytochemical	Source
1967	Roots	Piperlongumine and piperlonguminine have been isolated.	Chatterjee et al
2005	Fruit	Piperine: A alkaloid was isolated and showed significant antidepressant like activity	Lee SA et al, Sharma et al.
2008	Leaf	Essential oil was analyzed: eugenol (33.11%), caryophyllene (9.29%), cinnamyl acetate (5.91%) and pinene (4.74%), whereas leaf oil rich in trans-nerolidol (19.08%), caryophyllene (12.25%), 3-heptene, 7-phenyl- (3.71%), benzyl benzoate (3.68%), caryophyllene oxide (3.62%) and β-elemene (3.28%).	Bhuiyan et al
2009	Whole plant	11 compounds were isolated from ethanolic extract: coumaperine, N-5-(4-hydroxy-3-methoxyphenyl)-2E-pentenoyl piperidine, piperolactam A, 1-[1-oxo-5 (3,4-methylenedioxyphenyl) -2E,4E-pentadienyl] -pirrolidine, 1-[1-oxo-5 (3,4-methylenedioxyphenyl) -2E-pentenyl] -pirrolidine, 1-[1-oxo-9 (3,4-methylene dioxyphenyl)-2E, 8E-nonadienyl] -pyrrolidine , (R)-(-) -turmerone, octahydro-4-hydroxy-3alpha-methyl-7-methylene-alpha-(1-methylethyl)-1H-indene-1-methanol, (+) -aphanamol I, bisdemethoxycurcumin, demethoxycurcumin.	Liu W et al
2010	Fruits	Tridecyl-dihydro-pcoumaarate,eicosanyl-(E)-p-coumarate and Z-12-octandecenoic –glycerol-monoester	Zaveri et al
2013	Fruits	Piperlongumamides A-C, together with 12 known ones were isolated	Yang et al

Pharmacological Review

Table 3.26: Pharmacological activities of *Piper longum*

Year	Plant Part	Pharmacological activity	Observation	Source
2000	Fruit	Antiulcer activity	Piperine reduced the indomethacin induced gastric ulcer in a dose dependent manner and decrease the volume of gastric juice, gastric	BAI-Yin F et al

Chapter 3　　　　　　　　　　　　　　　　　　　　　　　Literature Review

			acidity	
2003	Fruit	Hepatoprotective activity	Ethanolic extract and butanolic fraction showed significant Hepatoprotective activity when compared with control Liv-52.	Jalalpure et al
2004	Fruit	Anticancer activity and Immunomodulatory activity	Alcoholic extracts of fruits and piperine showed toxic effect against Dalton's lymphoma ascites (DLA) and also increase significantly total WBC count	Sunila et al
2005	Fruit	Antidepressant activity	Piperine: A alkaloid was isolated and showed significant antidepressant like activity by inhibiting Mono amino oxidase enzyme	Lee SA et al
2009	Fruit	Anti-inflammatory activity	Dried's Fruit oil showed good anti-inflammatory effect in carrageenan-induced rat paw edema.	Kumar et al
2013, 2011	Root	Antidiabetic activity, antioxidant, Anti-hyperlipidemia	Aqueous extract of roots showed significant decrease in Fasting blood glucose level and also corrected diabetic dyslipidemia in rats. Ethanolic extract of fruits showed effective reduction in blood glucose level in STZ induced diabetic rats.	Nabi et al Kumar et al
2013	Areial	Antimicrobial activity	Acetone, petroleum ether and ethanol extracts of all the parts were tested against certain bacterial strains of E.coli, Steptococcusfaecalis, Steptococcuspyogens and Salmonella paratyphia and showed significant zone of inhibition.	Sindhu et al

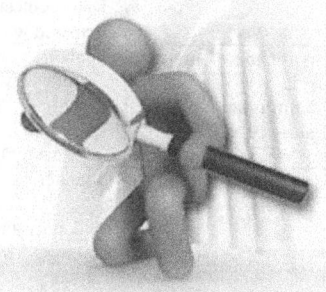

CHAPTER-4
Material and methods

4.1 PHASE-I

4.1.1 Procurement and Authentication of Plant material.

All parts of 10 medicinal plants were collected in the month of July to October from the village of Barabanki district and local market Lucknow, Uttar Pradesh India.

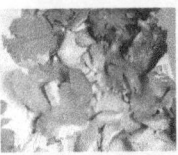 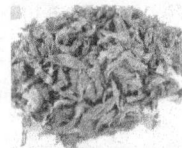

The dried plant materials were authentified at National Botanical Research Institute (NBRI) Lucknow. The voucher specimen no. NBRI-SOP-202 of the plants was deposited at the Department of Pharmacy SITM Barabanki for further reference. All the plant material were properly washed, dried under shade and powered each drug were prepared.

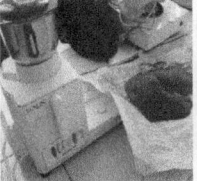 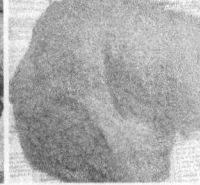

4.1.2 Quality assessment/Physiochemical evaluation of plant materials

Quality assessment of plant materials was done as per the standard procedure of Ayurvedic Pharmacopeia of India. Different parameters were tested with the methods describe in API.

1) **Foreign organic matter**: According to Ayurvedic Pharmacopeia of India, Foreign matter is described as any material that consist of part of organ or organ part from which the drug is derived. The plant should be free from any foreign particle like dust, insects, faecal matter etc. The percentage of foreign matter should not be more than the limit prescribed in monograph. There should not be any contamination in drug material used for developing the polyherbal formulation.

Procedure: 100-500 gm of plant materials were weighed and spread as a thin layer and was inspected first with naked eyes and then with the use of lens (6x). All the foreign matter were separated, weighed and percentage was calculated.

2) **Determination of Total ash value:** 3 gm of dried powered sample was weighed in silica dish and was incinerated at a temperature not exceeding 450°C until it get free from carbon. The incinerated material was cooled, weighed and percentage of ash was calculated with reference to air dried drug.

3) **Determination of Acid insoluble ash value**: Ash obtained was boiled with 25 ml of dil. Hydrochloric acid for 5 minutes filtered and insoluble matter was collected in crucible and washed with hot water and ignited till constant weight. The percentage of acid insoluble ash was calculated with respect to air dried drug.

4) **Determination of Water soluble ash**: Ash obtained (in determination of total ash value) was boiled with 25 ml of water for 5 minutes filtered it and insoluble matter was washed with hot water ignited till constant weight. The weight of insoluble matter was subtracted from the weight of the total ash and percentage was calculated with reference to air dried drug.

5) **Determination of Alcohol soluble extractive value**: 5gm of powdered drug was macerated with 100 ml of alcohol in cork fitted conical flask. Solution was shaken frequently for 6 hrs. and was allowed to stand for 18 hrs. After 18 hr. content was filtered and 25 ml of filtrate was evaporated to dryness in a shallow dish at 105°C to constant weight and percentage of alcohol soluble extractives was calculated with reference to air dried drug.

6) **Determination of water-soluble extractives:** 5gm of powdered drug was macerated with 100 ml of water in cork fitted conical flask. Solution was shaken frequently for 6 hrs. and was allowed to stand for 18 hrs. After 18 hr. content was filtered and 25 ml of filtrate was evaporated to dryness in a shallow dish at 105°C to constant weight and percentage of water soluble extractives was calculated with reference to air dried drug.

The data generated in respect of above findings will be used as in-house standards.

4.2 PHASE-II

4.2.1 Preparation of hydro alcoholic extracts

All the plant materials were extracted separately with ethanol (40:60) in soxhlet apparatus, the solvent was removed by distillation and concentrated extract was dried under vacuum. The percentage yield of each extract was calculated.

Chapter 4

Extraction Procedure

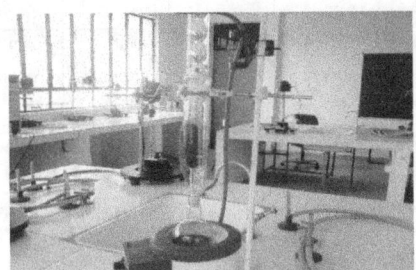

Figure 4.1: Extraction by using Soxhlet apparatus

4.2.2 Preliminary Phyto-chemical screening of hydro alcoholic plant extracts.

Crude extract of plants were subjected to different chemical tests to detect the presence of various phytochemical constituents as per procedure adopted in literature by Madhav et al (2011) and Saha et al (2011). The details are incorporated below in the following table. Results of the entire chemical test are discussed in Chapter 5 Results

Table 4.1: Preliminary Phytochemical screening of Plants

Chemical constituent	Name of Chemical test	Procedure	*Annona squamosa*	*Morus alba*	*Nelumbo nucifera*	*Psidium guajava*	*Coccinia indica*
Alkaloids	Mayer's reagent test	Extract+dil. HCl+3ml Mayer's reagent	Yellow precipitate obtained	Yellow precipitate obtained	Yellow precipitate obtained	No Yellow ppt. obtained	Yellow precipitate obtained
	Dragendroff reagent test	Extract+dil HCl+3ml Dragendroff reagent	Reddish brown ppt.	Reddish brown ppt.	Reddish brown ppt.	Reddish brown ppt.	Reddish brown ppt.
Glycosides	Legal's test	Extract+ 10%NaOH +sodium	Blue colour appeared	Blue color appeared	Blue colour appeared	Blue colour appeared	Blue color appeared

		nitroprusside					
Saponins	Foam test	Extract+water+shaken vigorously	Persistent Foam appeared	Foam appeared	Foam appeared	Foam appeared	Foam appeared
Flavonoids	Lead acetate test	Extract + solution of lead acetate+	Yellow ppt. formed	Yellow ppt. formed	Yellow ppt. formed	Yellow ppt. formed	Yellow ppt. formed
Carbohydrates	Fehling's Test	1 ml Fehling A+1ml Fehling mixed and boiled for minute+	Brick red ppt.formed	Brick red ppt.formed	Brick red ppt.formed	Brick red ppt.formed	Brick red ppt.formed
Steroids	Salkowski test	Extract(2ml)+2ml chloroform +2ml conc.H_2SO_4 +Shaken	Chloroform layer turn red and acid layer green	Chloroform layer turn red and acid layer green	No red chloroform layer formed	Chloroform layer turn red and acid layer green	No red chloroform layer formed
Tannins & Phenolic compounds	$FeCl_3$ test	Extract+5% $FeCl_3$	Deep blue coloured	Deep blue coloured	No Deep blue coloured	Deep blue coloured	No Deep blue colour appeared

Table 4.2: Preliminary Phytochemical screening of Plants

Chemical constituent	Name of Chemical test	Procedure	*Momordica charantia*	*Syzium cumini*	*Gymnea sylvestre*	*Pterocarpus marsupium*	*Piper longum*
Alkaloids	Mayer's reagent test	Extract+dil. HCl+3ml Mayer's reagent	Yellow ppt. obtained	Yellow ppt. obtained	White yellowish ppt. obtained	Yellow ppt. obtained	Yellow ppt. obtained

	Dragendroff reagent test	Extract+dil HCl+3ml Dragendroff reagent	Reddish brown ppt.	Reddish brown ppt.	Reddish brown ppt.	Reddish brown ppt.	Reddish ppt. obtained
Glycosides	Legal's test	Extract+ 10%NaOH +sodium nitroprusside	Blue colour appeared	Blue colour appeared	Blue colour appeared	Blue colour appeared	Blue colour appeared
Saponins	Foam test	Extract+water+shaken vigorously	Persistent Foam appeared	Persistent Foam appeared	Frothing appears	Frothing appears	Frothing appears
Flavonoids	Lead acetate test	Extract + solution of lead acetate	Yellow ppt. formed	Yellow ppt. formed	Yellow ppt. formed	Yellow ppt. formed	Yellow ppt. formed
Carbohydrates	Fehling's Test	1 ml Fehling A+1ml Fehling mixed and boiled for minute+	Brick red ppt.formed	No Brick red ppt.formed	Red-Orange ppt. obtained	Red-Orange ppt. obtained	Red-Orange ppt. obtained
Steroids	Salkowski test	Extract(2ml)+2 ml chloroform+2ml conc.H_2SO_4 +Shaken	Chloroform layer turn red and acid layer green	Chloroform layer turn red and acid layer green	Red colour in the lower layer Obtained	Red colour in the lower layer Obtained	Red colour in the lower layer Obtained
Tannins & Phenolic compounds	$FeCl_3$ test	Extract+5% $FeCl_3$	No deep blue coloured	Deep blue coloured	Blue back colour appeared	Deep blue coloured	No deep blue coloured

4.3 PHASE-III
4.3.1 Design and Development of Polyherbal Formulations.

From the extracts of ten plants six formulations have been made by blending the extracts in such a way so that it covers most of targeted sites in body to decrease the blood glucose level for their anti-diabetic action. For 3 formulations (A,B,C) quantity of doses used in developing the formulation was calculated on the basis of therapeutic doses reported in literatures and for next three formulations equal quantity of doses of extracts was used in developing the polyherbal formulations.

Table 4.3: Design of Polyherbal formulations by amalgamation of traditional and emerging anti-diabetic plant extracts

Formulation	Plant added	Part Used	Quantity (mg)	Reference for Reported mode of action of plant
A	Annona squamosa	Leaves	50	Gupta et al (2005)
	Morus alba	Leaves	170	Habeeb et al (2012) ; Sudha et al (2011)
	Coccinia indica	Leaves	50	Shibib et al (1993);Hossain et al (1992)
	Nelumbo nucifera	Leaves	50	Huralikuppi et al (1991)
	Gymnea sylvestre	Leaves	130	Kanetkar et al (2007); Baskaranet al (1990)
	Piper longum	Fruits	50	Patil et al (2011); Myung Joo et al (2009)
B	Annona squamosa	Leaves	60	Gupta et al (2005)
	Morus alba	Leaves	180	Habeeb et al (2012) ; Sudha et al (2011)
	Nelumbo nucifera	Leaves	50	Huralikuppi et al (1991)
	Syzium cumini	Seeds	110	Sudha et al (2011)
	Pterocarpus marsupium	Heartwood	90	Chakravarty et al (1980)
C	Nelumbo nucifera	Leaves	60	Huralikuppi et al (1991)
	Gymnea sylvestre	Leaves	210	Kanetkar et al (2007); Baskaranet al (1990)
	Psidium guajava	Leaves	120	
	Momordica charantia	Fruits	60	Sudha et al (2011)
	Piper longum	Fruits	50	Shibib et al (1993) Patil et al (2011) ; Myung Joo et al,(2009)

Table 4.4: Design of Polyherbal formulations (with equal doses of each extract)

Formulation	Plant added	Part Used	Quantity (mg)	Reported mode of action for plant
D	Annona squamosa	Leaves	100	Gupta et al (2005)
	Morus alba	Leaves	100	Habeeb et al (2012), Sudha et al (2011)
	Nelumbo nucifera	Leaves	100	Huralikuppi et al (1991)
	Psidium guajava	Leaves	100	Sudha et al (2011)
	Piper longum	Fruits	100	Patil et al (2011), Myung Joo et al (2009)
E	Gymnea sylvestre	Leaves	100	Kanetkar et al(2007), Baskaranetal(1990)
	Momordica charantia	Fruit	100	Shibib et al (1993)
	Pterocarpus marsupium	Heartwood	100	Chakravarty et al (1980)
		Seeds	100	Sudha et al (2011)
	Syzium cumini	Fruits	100	Patil et al (2011), Myung Joo et al (2009)
	Piper longum			
F	Annona squamosa	Leaves	100	Gupta et al (2005)
	Morus alba	Leaves	100	Habeeb et al (2012), Sudha et al (2011)
	Pterocarpus marsupium	Heartwood	100	Chakravarty et al (1980)
		Leaves	100	Kanetkar et al(2007), Baskaranet al(1990)
	Gymnea sylvestre	Fruits	100	Patil et al(2011), Myung Joo et al (2009)
	Piper longum			

4.4 PHASE-IV

4.4.1 Acute toxicity study of polyherbal formulation as per OECD guidelines

4.4.1.1 Preparation of Formulations

For dosing 100 ml of each formulation was prepared by dissolving 5 gm of formulation in 100 ml of distilled water (so that 1 ml contain 50 mg of drug).

4.4.1.2 Experimental Animals

For experimental study, albino wistar rats (150-200g) with same age group of either sex were obtained from Indian Institute of Toxicological Research (IITR) Lucknow. Animals were accommodated in polypropylene cages at a surrounding temperature of 25-30 °C and relative humidity was 45-55 % with a 12 hr. each of dark and light cycle in an animal house of King George Medical College (CSMMU) Lucknow. Animals were fed pellet diet and water *ad libitum*. The study protocol was approved by Institutional Animal ethical committee of King George Medical College Lucknow as per the guidelines of Control and Supervision of Experiments on Animals (CPCSEA) Ministry of Environment and Forests, Government of India

4.4.1.3 Acute toxicity study of Polyherbal formulations

Acute toxicity studies were carried out in adult female albino rats weighing between 130-180g by Acute Oral Toxicity method of OECD Guideline No 423. They were administered (orally) with varying doses (250, 500, 1000 and 2000 mg/kg body weight) for each of six formulations. Animals were divided into 5 groups of three animals each and were acclimatized for 5 days. Prior to dosing animals were kept fasted overnight and next day each formulation were administered orally at a dose level of 250, 500, 1000 and 2000 mg / kg b.wt. The Rats were observed for clinical signs of toxicity continuously for 2 hours and occasionally for further 4 hours for general behavioral and finally for any mortality after 24 hours till 14 days. No mortality was observed during a time period of 14 days.

4.5 PHASE-V

4.5.1 Oral glucose tolerance test of all formulations

4.5.1.1 Selection of dose

Two dose level were chosen in such a way that one dose was approximately one-tenth of the maximum dose used during the acute toxicity studies, second dose was the twice that of one-tenth dose (200mg/kg, 400mg/kg b. wt)

4.5.1.2 Initial Screening of all the Polyherbal Formulations for Anti-hyperglycemic activity (Oral Glucose Tolerance Test)

All the formulations A, B, C, D, E and F were screened for anti-hyperglycemic activity to get the information on their efficacy so that the formulation which is not effective could be modified. All the 6 formulations were analyzed for anti-hyperglycemic activity in normal healthy rats by conducting Oral Glucose Tolerance Test (OGTT). Initial testing was carried out at different dose levels of all 6 formulations (200 and 400 mg/kg b.wt). Overnight fasted rats were weighed and divided in to fourteen groups with 5 rats in each group for each formulation as given below. After 30 minutes, rats of all groups were loaded orally with glucose 2g/kg b.wt. Blood glucose level was determined by glucometer before and at 30 min, 60 min, 120 min, 150 min and 180 min after loading with glucose.

Group Design for OGTT study

- Group I – Normal Control treated with vehicle i.e (2ml/kg) distilled water
- Group II- Standard given Glibenclamide (5mg/b.wt)
- Group III- treated orally with F-A 200 mg/kg b.wt.
- Group IV- treated orally with F-A 400 mg/kg b.wt.
- Group V- treated orally with F-B 200 mg/kg b.wt.
- Group VI- treated orally with F-B 400 mg/kg b.wt.
- Group VII- treated orally with F-C 200 mg/kg b.wt.
- Group VIII- treated orally with F-C 400 mg/kg b.wt.
- Group IX- treated orally with F-D 200 mg/kg b.wt.
- Group X- treated orally with F-D 400 mg/kg b.wt.
- Group XI- treated orally with F-E 200 mg/kg b.wt.
- Group XII- treated orally with F-E 400 mg/kg b.wt.

- Group XIII- treated orally with F-F 200 mg/kg b.wt.
- Group XIV- treated orally with F-F 400 mg/kg b.wt.

4.6 PHASE-VI

4.6.1 Antidiabetic activity

4.6.1.1 Study protocol: Induction of diabetes and experimental study

Diabetes was induced in rats by intra-peritoneal injection of Streptozotocin (60 mg/kg b.wt) which was dissolved in normal saline. After 72 hrs. of Streptozotocin administration blood glucose level was measured by glucometer (Escencia entrust, Bayer health care) to confirm diabetes. Blood samples were drawn by picking the rat tail. The diabetic rats with blood glucose levels ≥ 250 mg/dl were selected for the studies.

After 72 hr. of STZ injection animal with BGL $\geq$ 250 mg/dl were divided into different groups (with 5 animals each) for anti-diabetic study of Formulations. Following groups were prepared:

- Group I –Normal control (given distilled water)
- Group II-Negative control (treated with STZ 60 mg/kg b.wt i.p)
- Group III-Standard (Treated with Glibenclamide 5mg/kg b.wt after 3rd day of STZ injection)
- Group IV-Treated orally with Formulation A with dose of 200 mg/kg b.wt after 3rd day of STZ injection
- Group V- Treated orally with Formulation A dose of 400 mg/kg b.wt after 3rd day of STZ injection
- Group VI-Treated orally with Formulation B with dose of 200 mg/kg b.wt after 3rd day of STZ injection
- Group VII- Treated orally with Formulation B with dose of 400 mg/kg b.wt after 3rd day of STZ injection

- Group VIII-Treated orally with Formulation C with dose of 200 mg/kg b.wt after 3rd day of STZ injection
- Group IX- Treated orally with Formulation C with dose of 400 mg/kg b.wt after 3rd day of STZ injection
- Group X-Treated orally with Formulation D with dose of 200 mg/kg b.wt after 3rd day of STZ injection
- Group XI-Treated orally with Formulation D with dose of 400 mg/kg b.wt after 3rd day of STZ injection
- Group XII-Treated orally with Formulation E with dose of 200 mg/kg b.wt after 3rd day of STZ injection
- Group XIII-Treated orally with Formulation E with dose of 400 mg/kg b.wt after 3rd day of STZ injection
- Group XIV-Treated orally with Formulation F with dose of 200 mg/kg b.wt after 3rd day of STZ injection
- Group XV-Treated orally with Formulation F with dose of 400 mg/kg b.wt after 3rd day of STZ injection

Study was conducted for 15 days. Treatment was started from 3rd day. Standard drug and Formulations given daily for 15 days and blood glucose levels were measured with the help of Glucometer (Ascensia ENTRUST, Bayer Health Care) on 3rd day (assume as 0 hrs.), after 3 hrs., 5th day, 10th day and 15th day of experiment. Blood sample was taken by picking the rat tail vein and for the measurement of other biochemical parameters blood sample was withdrawn from retro-orbital plexus of rats. Hussain et al (2011)

4.6.2 Assessment of Biochemical parameters

At the end of 15 day of experiment, 2-4 ml blood sample was withdrawnfrom retro-orbital plexus of rats and centrifuged at the 5000 rpm for 15-20 min; serum was separated and was taken out with the help of syringe. Serum of rats was used for the analysis of other biochemical parameters through Auto analyzer

Following biochemical parameters were analysed:

a)   Total Cholesterol(TC)
b)   Total Triglycerides (TG)
c)   High Density Lipoprotein (HDL)
d)   Low Density Lipoprotein (LDL)
e)   Urea
f)   Creatinine
g)   Serum Glutamate Oxaloacetic acid Transferase (SGOT)
h)   Serum Glutamate Pyruvate Transferase (SGPT)

The data were analysed by two-way ANOVA and results are expressed as Mean±S.E

4.7 PHASE VII

4.7.1 Quality control/Standardization of Polyherbal formulations

Herbal drug standardization is necessary to control the batch to batch variations in the product However the standardization of herbal medicine is a challenging task as herbal medicines contain number of active ingredient hence it is very difficult to establish parameter for quality control, even for most of the herbal active ingredient no official standards procedures and limits of different physicochemical parameters are available. Pattanayak et al (2011) and Pandey et al (2011) in their study reveal that there are three main pharmacopeial definitions are included in term QUALITY CONTROL

a)   Identity of herb
b)   purity of herb and
c)   content of active constituents

The most difficult is to assess the contents of herbal medicine because most of the active ingredients are unknown in herbal formulation however Rasheed et al (2012) in their review evidently point out that sometimes marker can be used with HPTLC which can ensure the concentration of corresponding ingredients in formulations. CCRAS laboratory guide also gives the detailed description of standardization of Ayurvedic herbal formulations which help in establishing the in house standardized parameters for polyherbal formulations.

4.7.1.1 HPTLC fingerprinting analysis of all the polyherbal combinations

It is used for the identification, purity determination and strength determination of polyherbal formulation and hence helps in developing and fixing the standards for it. To ensure the availability of different active constituents in polyherbal formulation, the HPTLC study of these in-house polyherbal formulations were carried out with the use of following standard/ marker compounds.

- Quercetin
- Rutin
- Stigmasterol
- Gallic acid
- Ellagic acid
- Catechin
- Epicatechin and
- Piperine

Following instruments were used for HPTLC profiling of in-house polyherbal formulations:

DESAGA Sarstedt Gruppe system (ProQuant 1.6 version software) with Automatic TLC applicator (as an application mode) and Densitometer CD 60 (for scanning of spots) were used. Pre-coated Silica gel 60 F 254 Plates were used to develop the TLC in Twin trough TLC Chamber.

Chromatographic conditions:

Stationary phase: Silica gel 60 F 254 Plates

Mobile Phase: Toluene: EAA (17:3.5 % v/v)

TLC chamber saturation time was 30 min.

Temperature $25 \pm 2\,°C$ and relative humidity 40 %

Procedure: Different mobile phases were referred as discussed by Wagner in "Plant Drug Analysis" to get the best separations of plant compounds. Toluene: EAA (17:3.5 % v/v) combination emerged as best mobile phase to develop the TLC plates. For spotting 10 μl of each sample and standard were applied on TLC plates. TLC Plates were then allowed to develop in mobile phase (Toluene: EAA (17:3.5 % v/v)) until it reaches one-fourth of TLC plate in Twin trough TLC Chamber. The spots were dried and scanned under the U.V range of 366 nm and 254 nm.

4.7.1.2 Safety assessment

Safety evaluation is one of the important parameter of herbal drug standardization. For the safety assessment the toxicity of formulation should be evaluated. Deamination of Acute oral toxicity is considered as a first step to develop the therapeutic dose. Heavy metal content determination is another safety assessment parameter.

4.7.1.2.1 Heavy Metal Content Determination by Atomic Absorption Spectroscopy as adopted by Bushra et al 2011 and Suganya et al (2012)

Heavy metal content determination (Mercury, Lead, Arsenic and Cadmium) was done by Atomic Absorption Spectroscopy at Biotech Park Lucknow

4.7.1.2.2 Microbial load by plate count method

Microbial load (bacteria and fungi) was determined by plate count method as per Ayurvedic Pharmacopeia of India Vol II 2.4.1 at Biotech Park Lucknow.

A) For Bacteria:

✓ 10 petridish (9 to 10 cm diameter) were used for bacteria count. All the Petri dishes were washed properly and autoclaved at 120 ° C for 15 min.

✓ A mixture of 1 ml of the pretreated preparation and about 15 ml of liquefied casein soya bean digest agar medium (temp. not more than 45°) was added in each petri dish.

✓ Pretreated preparation was spread on the surface of solidified medium in a petri dish of the same diameter.

- ✓ Pretreated preparation was diluted so that a colony count should not more than 300.
- ✓ All the Petri-dishes were incubated at 30-35°C for 5 days. After 5 days numbers of colonies were counted.

B) For Fungi:

- ✓ Sabouraud dextrose agar is used with antibiotics in place of casein soyabean digest agar for the microbial count of fungi.
- ✓ Plates were incubated at 20 to 25°C for 5 days and colonies were counted.

CHAPTER-5

Results and Observations

5.1 Physiochemical evaluation of plant materials:

It was observed that all physicochemical evaluation parameters contain i.e. foreign organic matter, Total ash, Acid insoluble ash, Alcohol extractive and water-soluble extractives of plant drug was found to be within Ayurvedic pharmacopeia limits. Foreign organic matter was found to be 0.001% in *Momordica charantia* can be considered as nil as given in API. For some of the emerging plant drugs *Psidium guajava, Annona squamosa, Morus alba* and *Nelumbo nucifera* are not included in Ayurvedic Pharmacopeia of India, quality control standards of physicochemical parameters are developed for this study. Each value represents an average of data obtained from samples collected from different localities. The data generated here will be used as in-house standards. (*) showed that API limits of physicochemical parameters these emerging plants are not given in Ayurvedic Pharmacopeia of India (table 5.1 and 5.2).

Table 5.1: Results of Physico-chemical evaluation of the plant material

Parameter	*Momordica charantia*		*Syzygium cumini*		*Pterocarpus marsupium*		*Gymnea sylvestre*		*Piper longum*	
	Obtained Value	API Limit	Obtained Value	API Limit	Obtained Value	API Limit	Obtained Value	API Limit	Obtained Value	API limit
Foreign organic matter	0.001%	NIL	1.85±.05	NMT2%	1.76±01	NMT 2%	1.07±0.06	NMT2%	1.76±0.23	NMT 2%
Total ash value	3.47±.23	NMT5%	4.32±.22	NMT5%	1.57±.25	NMT 2%	11.03±0.01	NMT12%	1.68±0.02	NMT 7%
Acid insoluble ash value	0.45±.01	NMT0.6%	1.34±.25	NMT2%	0.25±.03	NMT 0.5%	1.03±.042	NMT2%	0.35±0.012	NMT0.5%
Alcohol extractive value	8.38±0.72	NLT6%	14.68.±54	NLT12%	9.56±.36	NLT 7%	9.45±0.56	NLT7%	7.04±0.36	NLT 5%
Water soluble extractive value	30.76±0.51	NMT28%	25.42±.76	NLT 23%	7.42±.74	NLT 5%	30.45±.043	NLT28%	9.65±0.43	NLT7%

(NMT-Not more than, NLT –Not less than)

Table 5.2: Results of Physicochemical evaluation of the plant material

Parameters	Coccinia indica		Nelumbo nucifera*	Psidium guajava*	Morus alba*	Annona squamosa*
	Obtained Value	API limit Value	Obtained Value	Obtained Value	Obtained Value	Obtained Value
Foreign organic matter	1.42 ±.03	NMT2%	1.94±.21	1.76±.31	1.82±.22	1.66±.54
Total ash value	1.53 ±21	NMT 2%	9.03±.02	8.01±.50	13.83±.67	8.92±0.53
Acid insoluble ash value	1.29±.32	NMT 2%	1.28+.23	1.67±0.52	1.12±0.37	1.21±0.04
Alcohol extractive value	5.63 ±.49	NLT 3%	2.12±.04	6.05±0.05	5.09±0.03	19.08± 0.87
Water soluble extractive value	16.67±.42	NLT14%	16.45±.54	12.67±0.32	14.84±0.45	20.94±0.25

(NMT-Not more than, NLT –Not less than)

5.2 Percentage yield of all the hydro-alcoholic plant extracts

The percentage yields of all hydro alcoholic plant extract are given in table 5.3.

Table 5.3: Percentage yield of hydro-alcoholic plant extracts

Name of Plant Drug	Powdered plant drug (gm)	Solvent used EtOH:H_2O (40:60)	% yield
Psidium guajava	100gm	800ml	15.29%
Annona squamosa	100gm	800ml	11.6 %
Morus alba	100gm	800ml	25%
Syzygium cumini	100gm	800ml	15.25%
Nelumbo nucifera	100gm	800ml	12.89%
Coccinia indica	100gm	800 ml	9.70%
Momordica charantia	100gm	800ml	1.46%
Piper longum	100gm	800ml	12.30%
Gymnea sylvestre	100gm	800ml	17.58%
Pterocarpus marsupium	100gm	800ml	10.20%

5.3 Preliminary Phytochemical screening of hydro alcoholic plant extracts

Results of phytochemical screening are shown in table 5.4. It was found that *Annona squamosa* and *Morus alba* contain all tested phytochemical compounds.

Table 5.4: Results of Preliminary Phytochemical screening of Plants

Chemical tests	Momordica charantia	Morus alba	Psidium guajava	Nelumbo nucifera	Piper longum
Alkaloids	+	+	-	+	+
Glycosides	+	+	+	+	+
Flavonoids	+	+	+	+	+
Saponins	+	+	+	+	+
Carbohydrates	+	+	+	+	+
Phenolic compounds and tannins	-	+	+	-	-
Steroids	+	+	+	-	+

Table 5.5: Results of Preliminary Phytochemical screening of Plants

Chemical tests	Annona squamosa	Syzium cumini	Coccinia indica	Pterocarpus Marsupium	Gymnea sylvestre
Alkaloids	+	+	+	+	+
Glycosides	+	+	+	+	+
Flavonoids	+	++	+	+	+
Saponins	+	+	+	+	+
Tannins and Phenolic compounds	+	++	-	+	+
Carbohydrate	+	-	-	+	+
Steroids	+	+	-	+	+

(+) sign indicated the presence and (--) sign indicated the absence of phytochemicals.

5.4 Acute toxicity study of polyherbal formulation

STZ-induced diabetic rats treated with all six formulations did not show any discernible change in behaviour up to the dose level of 2000 mg/kg body weight. No sign of mortality was observed during the observation of 14 days (table: 5.6 to 5.11).

Table 5.6: Results of Toxicity study of Formulation A

Group	No of rats	Wt. of rats (gm)	Dose of Formulation	Calculated dose (ml)	No. of dead animals
I	3	150.23	250 mg/kg b.wt	0.75	Nil
		148.79		0.74	
		150.12		0.75	
II	3	151.40	500mg/kg b.wt	1.51	Nil
		145.62		1.45	
		156.01		1.56	
III	3	150.92	1000 mg/kg b.wt	3.01	Nil
		150.12		3.00	
		152.34		3.04	
IV	3	155.03	2000 mg/kg b.wt	6.20	Nil
		142.34		5.69	
		145.73		5.82	

Table 5.7: Results of Toxicity study of Formulation B

Group	No of rats	Wt. of rats (gm)	Dose of Formulation	Calculated dose(ml)	No. of dead animals
I	3	160.31	250 mg/kg b.wt	0.80	Nil
		148.02		0.74	
		153.12		0.76	
II	3	151.01	500mg/kg b.wt	1.51	Nil
		149.67		1.49	
		158.02		1.58	
III	3	164.32	1000 mg/kg b.wt	3.28	Nil
		160.43		3.20	
		157.02		3.14	
IV	3	153.47	2000 mg/kg b.wt	6.13	Nil
		160.05		6.40	
		152.01		6.08	

Table 5.8: Results of Toxicity study of Formulation C

Group	No of rats	Wt. of rats (gm)	Dose of Formulation	Calculated dose(ml)	No. of dead animals
I	3	156.73	250 mg/kg b.wt	0.78	Nil
		150.98		0.75	
		154.76		0.77	
II	3	151.89	500mg/kg b.wt	1.51	Nil
		153.90		1.53	
		178.87		1.78	
III	3	156.32	1000 mg/kg b.wt	3.12	Nil
		167.54		3.35	
		159.04		3.18	
IV	3	176.34	2000 mg/kg b.wt	7.05	Nil
		160.09		6.40	
		153.17		6.12	

Table: 5.9: Results of Toxicity study of formulation D

Group	No of rats	Wt. of rats (gm.)	Dose of Formulation	Calculated dose (ml)	No. of dead animals
I	3	164.78	250 mg/kg b.wt	0.82	Nil
		174.32		0.87	
		159.87		0.79	
II	3	165.09	500mg/kg b.wt	1.65	Nil
		187.32		1.87	
		163.17		1.63	
III	3	173.98	1000 mg/kg b.wt	3.47	Nil
		159.98		3.19	
		166.65		3.33	
IV	3	167.63	2000 mg/kg b.wt	6.70	Nil
		170.54		6.82	
		168.71		6.74	

Table: 5.10: Results of Toxicity study of formulation E

Group	No of rats	Wt. of rats (gm.)	Dose of Formulation	Calculated dose(ml)	No. of dead animals
I	3	159.78	250 mg/kg b.wt	0.79	Nil
		164.07		0.82	
		172.39		0.86	
II	3	193.27	500mg/kg b.wt	1.93	Nil
		187.93		1.87	
		176.56		1.76	
III	3	194.76	1000 mg/kg b.wt	3.89	Nil
		186.45		3.72	
		159.67		3.19	
IV	3	188.42	2000 mg/kg b.wt	7.53	Nil
		179.57		7.18	
		192.67		7.70	

Table: 5.11: Results of Toxicity study of formulation F

Group	No of rats	Wt. of rats (gm.)	Dose of Formulation	Calculated dose(ml)	No. of dead animals
I	3	163.71	250 mg/kg b.wt	0.81	Nil
		171.73		0.85	
		175.21		0.87	
II	3	162.58	500mg/kg b.wt	1.62	Nil
		157.75		1.57	
		183.53		1.83	
III	3	161.43	1000 mg/kg b.wt	3.22	Nil
		175.09		3.50	
		182.76		3.65	
IV	3	181.79	2000 mg/kg b.wt	7.27	Nil
		186.90		7.40	
		191.72		7.60	

5.5 Oral glucose tolerance test

At 30 min after the administration of 2gm/kg glucose orally, the plasma glucose level is significantly increased and the blood glucose level decreases gradually with the administration of formulations. Results are given in table: 5.12 and results expressed in Mean ± SD in table 5.13.

Table 5.12: Results of Oral glucose tolerance test

Group	Treatment	No.of rats	Weight of rats (gm)	Dose	Cal. dose (ml)	Fasting BGL mg/dl	After loading with glucose 2g/kg b.wt -Oral Glucose Tolerance Test				
							30 min	60 min	120 min	150 min	180 min
I	Control	5	153.12	2ml/kg b.wt	0.30	69	110	120	128	130	122
			150.02		0.30	75	99	110	118	127	123
			156.78		0.31	70	105	117	120	135	129
			160.32		0.32	60	95	120	127	142	135
			152.48		0.30	58	90	115	122	135	130
II	Glibenclamide	5	149.85	5mg/kg b.wt	1.48	58	96	76	65	58	53
			151.25		1.5	51	106	88	76	63	59
			168.74		1.64	60	104	89	79	63	57
			168.53		1.64	65	99	80	73	66	60
			160.01		1.6	68	117	97	80	70	65
III a	F-A	5	168.45	200mg/ kg b.wt	0.67	73	95	89	84	80	78
			163.75		0.65	70	110	102	95	89	85
			155.32		0.62	66	120	111	99	89	84
			150.43		0.60	68	103	85	79	73	68
			150.01		0.59	66	100	91	86	62	58
III b	F-A	5	169.45	400 mg /kg b.wt	1.35	74	105	92	85	80	78
			149.55		1.19	60	82	78	74	66	60
			150.67		1.20	59	95	88	79	72	68
			158.66		1.26	62	102	90	84	80	76
			160.13		1.28	61	110	101	90	87	80
IV a	F-B	5	168.55	200	0.67	61	98	82	76	73	70

			158.23	mg/kg b.wt	0.63	67	112	104	94	88	79
			155.11		0.62	69	106	98	92	88	84
			153.45		0.61						
			151.02		0.60	72	117	107	95	86	75
						59	95	84	79	74	70
IV b	F-B	5	150.11	400 mg/kg b.wt	1.2	65	81	76	70	60	58
			150.87		1.19	73	99	83	79	74	66
			155.88		1.24						
			153.69		1.22	60	98	90	81	76	70
			162.12		1.29	62	100	90	82	78	73
						60	107	95	89	80	75
V a	F-C	5	168.32	200 mg/kg b.wt	0.67	65	106	96	86	78	69
			171.63		0.68	68	102	98	85	76	72
			150.90		0.60						
			151.55		0.60	69	108	94	86	80	74
			169.28		0.67	70	115	100	90	82	78
						73	98	90	84	78	75
V b	F-C	5	165.01	400 mg/kg b.wt	1.32	67	106	91	82	76	69
			158.83		1.27	65	100	86	78	68	64
			155.46		1.24						
			150.61		1.20	60	102	86	75	69	60
			169.41		1.35	59	100	83	72	66	58
						72	99	90	83	75	65
VI a	F-D	5	168.76	200mg/ kg b.wt	0.67	76	98	90	84	80	74
			168.34		0.67	88	119	111	104	98	90
			176.78		0.70	75	115	108	97	86	79
			159.23		0.63	69	99	88	79	72	68
			163.54		0.65	68	124	119	107	95	82
VI b	F-D	5	163.88	400 mg /kg.b.wt	1.31	72	100	94	89	80	78
			161.76		1.29	81	104	98	90	83	76
			157.21		1.25	78	99	92	84	79	71
			167.84		1.34	79	94	89	77	69	62
			173.43		1.38	61	99	101	90	87	80
VII a	F-E	5	179.08	200 mg/kg. b.wt	0.67	70	100	93	86	78	71
			177.57		0.71	69	112	107	98	86	77
			186.56		0.74	60	98	89	76	69	58
			183.64		0.73	81	118	109	95	87	75
			170.61		0.68	79	108	96	85	79	67
VII b	F-E	5	172.01	400 mg/kg	1.37	69	96	89	80	75	68

			161.73	b.wt	1.29	75	99	87	79	71	65
			159.45		1.27	68	102	96	88	79	70
			177.34		1.41	64	100	91	84	79	69
			163.63		1.30	73	109	99	87	76	67
						82	121	113	105	96	88
VIII a	F-F	5	181.98	200mg/kg b.wt	0.72	78	109	99	85	77	70
			177.65		0.71	85	111	103	94	86	76
			156.88		0.62	74	97	91	85	76	68
			161.44		0.64	70	99	90	86	78	75
			169.62		0.67						
						69	110	92	84	79	70
VIII b	F-F	5	172.41	400mg/kg b.wt	1.37	78	105	94	88	80	71
			186.11		1.48	75	103	92	85	79	70
			199.83		1.59	68	96	83	75	67	61
			188.94		1.51	79	99	90	83	75	65
			170.34		1.36						

Blood glucose levels are expressed as Mean±S.D

Table 5.13: Oral glucose tolerance test (Blood glucose level expressed in Mean± S.E)

GROUP	FASTING BGL	30 min	60 min	120 min	150 min	180 min
Control(2ml/kg)	66.4±3.20	99.8±3.54	116.4±1.86	123.8±1.94	133.8±2.55	127.8±2.39
Standard(5mg/kg)	60.4±2.94	104.4±3.61	86±3.67	74.6±2.69	64±1.97	58.8±1.95
F-A (200mg/kg)	68.6±1.32	105.6±4.34	95.6±4.77	88.6±3.66	78.6±5.12	74.6±5.13
(400 mg/kg)	63.2±2.74	98.8±4.85	89.8±3.69	82.4±2.73	77±3.63	72.4±3.70
F-B (200mg/kg)	65.6±2.44	107.2±4.55	95.±5.11	87.2±4.01	81.8±3.41	75.6±2.69
(400 mg/kg)	64±2.42	97±4.30	86.8±3.30	80.2±3.05	73.6±3.54	68.4±3.01
F-C (200mg/kg)	69±1.30	105.8±2.87	95.6±1.72	86.2±1.01	78.8±1.01	73.6±1.50
(400 mg/kg)	64.6±2.37	101.4±1.24	87.2±1.46	78±2.07	70.8±1.98	63.2±1.93
F-D (200mg/kg)	75.2±3.56	111±5.30	103.2±6.07	94.2±5.49	86.2±4.77	78.6±3.70

	(400 mg/kg)	74.2±3.62	99.2±1.59	94.8±2.13	86±2.51	79.6±2.99	73.4±3.21
F-E	(200mg/kg)	71.8±3.78	107.2±3.72	98.8±3.92	88±3.91	79.8±3.24	69.8±3.37
	(400mg/kg)	69.8±1.93	101.2±2.17	92.4±2.22	83.6±1.80	76±1.48	67.8±0.86
F-F	(200mg/kg)	77.8±2.69	107.4±4.35	99.2±4.22	91±3.88	82.6±3.78	75.4±3.48
	(400mg/kg)	73.8±2.26	102.6±2.42	90.2±1.90	83±2.16	76±2.40	67.4±1.91

Findings of OGTT study:

From the study it was predicted that all the six formulations possess Anti- hyperglycemic activity

For Formulation A

It was noticed that Formulation A with dose of 200 mg showed effective decrease in average blood glucose i.e. 11.2 % at 150 min and the average decrease in blood glucose level from 30 min to 180 min increases with increase in dose.

For Formulation B

It was found that Formulation B with dose of 200 mg/kg b.wt.showed effective decrease in blood glucose i.e. 12.4% at 180 min, dose 400 mg showed 10.5% at 60 min

For Formulation C

It was found that Formulation C with dose of 200 mg/kg b.wt showed maximum decrease in average blood glucose at 120 min, dose 400 mg/kg showed maximum decrease in BGL i.e. 14% at 60 min.

Formulation D (200 mg/kg) showed maximum decrease in average blood glucose level i.e. 8.81% at 180 min while with a dose of 400 mg/kg b.wt showed maximum decrease in BGL i.e. 9.28% at 120 min.

Formulation E (200 mg/kg) showed maximum oral glucose tolerance with decrease in average blood glucose level from 30 to 180 min.i.e. 35.07% with maximum decrease of 12.78% average BGL at 180 min.

Formulation E (400mg/kg): Its higher dose is less effective (33.00%) in decreasing the average BGL from 30 to 180 min however it showed maximum decrease in percentage of average blood glucose level i.e. 10.78% at 180min.

Formulation F (200 mg/kg) showed maximum decrease in percentage of average blood glucose level at 150 min i.e. 9.23%. Formulation F (400 mg/kg) showed maximum decrease in average BGL at 60 min i.e. 12.08%.

5.6 Antidiabetic activity

Wistar rats of either sex (150-180 g body weight) were used for this study. They were acclimatized and given proper diet. The experimental protocol was approved by CPCSEA from Institutional Animal Ethics Committee of Chhattrapati Sahuji Maharaj Medical University Lucknow (King George Medical College).

Results showed the significantly increase in blood glucose level in STZ treated diabetic rats. Glucose levels measured in blood of normal and experimental rats are given in table 5.14. Blood glucose levels were significantly decreased on daily oral administration with a slight decrease in body weight. On repeated administration of vehicle, 6 formulations and glibenclamide for 15 days, a sustained and significant ($P< 0.0001$) decrease in the average blood glucose level of diabetic rats was observed in all 6 formulations.

In FB (200 mg/kg and 400 mg/kg b.wt) showed maximum reduction in average blood glucose level to 61.2 % from 0th day to 15th day and 64.02% with maximum decrease in average blood glucose level to 67 mg/dl between 10th to 15th day and 61.4 mg/dl near to standard Glibenclamide (66.2%).whereas FA (200 mg/kg b.wt and 400 mg/kg b.wt) showed effective decrease in average Blood glucose level to 49.7% and 51.8 % between 0 day to 15th days with a maximum of 43.6 mg/dl and 54 mg/dl between 10 to 15 day. FC showed greater decrease in average Blood glucose level i.e. 59.8% at a dose of 200 mg/kg

b. wt as compared to dose of 400 mg/kg b.wt which showed 54.8% decrease in average blood glucose level from 0th to 15th day in diabetic rats as shown in table 5.15 (Results are expressed in Mean ± S.D)

Table 5.16 showed the average decrease in blood glucose level from 0 day to 15th day of all 6 formulations in comparison with Standard Glibenclamide.

In polyherbal formulation F-D at (200 mg/kg and 400 mg/kg) showed significantly decrease in the fasting blood serum glucose level i.e. 62.9% and 65.8% in the diabetic rats from 0th day to 15thday as shown in table 5.6.2. It was observed that throughout the study period of 15 days, dose 200 mg/kg showed maximum reduction (37.26%) in average BGL between 10th to 15day whereas dose 400 mg/kg showed maximum reduction (43.8%) between 10th to 15thdays. At the end of study, it was noticed that maximum reduction in Blood glucose level to 65.80 % was seen at 15thday with a dose of 400 mg/kg which was very much near (i.e. 66.2%) to standard drug glibenclamide 5m/kg.

From the results it was found that Polyherbal E (combination of only traditional antidiabetic plants) with dose of 400 mg/kg b.wt. showed maximum reduction (64.2 %) in average Blood glucose level from 0 day to day 15. F-E (400 mg) exhibited peak anti-hyperglycemic effect from day 10 to day 15 by reducing blood glucose level to 74.2 mg/dl which is higher than that of glibenclamide which showed peak anti-hyperglycemic effect around day 5 by reducing BGL to 58.6 mg/dl.

F-F (200 mg and 400 mg) showed onset of action around the same period i.e. around day 5. Polyherbal F exhibit peak anti-hyperglycemic effect between days10th to day 15th by reducing the blood glucose level to 60 mg/dl which is higher than standard glibenclamide.200 mg dose of polyherbal formulation F showed maximum reduction (56.2%) in average blood glucose level as compared to dose 400 mg.

5.7 Biochemical parameters (Table 5.17 – 5.26)

Serum TG, Total cholesterol, LDL-cholesterol were found to be increased significantly ($P<0.0001$) in STZ induced diabetic rats (shown in table: 5.17-5.24) as compared to non-diabetic control. HDL cholesterol was found to be significantly decreased in diabetic rats. Treatment with all formulations produces a significant reduction in elevated serum TG, TC, LDL-cholesterol level in diabetic rats. Maximum Increase in HDL level was found to be 57.12% (greater than standard) with a dose of F-D (400 mg/kg b. wt.) given in table: 5.25.

In Biochemical Parameters F-A (400 mg and 200 mg) showed maximum decrease in SGPT, Urea and LDL Cholesterol level i.e. 69.8%- near to glibenclamide, 43.36% and 39.6%.

F-B (200 mg) showed maximum increase in HDL between the 0 to 15th day to 45% as that of standard.

For formulation C no noticeable response was shown. In polyherbal D 400 mg showed maximum increase in HDL level to 57.12% and creatinine level to 57.46% which is greater than those of standard glibenclamide and all other formulations.

For polyherbal formulation E (200 mg) showed maximum reduction in urea 55.25% from 0 to 15 days as compare to other Polyherbals where F (200 mg) showed maximum increase in average percentage of HDL i.e. 45.05% which is comparable to standard 45.4%.

Polyherbal E (200 mg and 400 mg) showed an approximately equal increase in average percentage of HDL (i.e. 34.12 and 34.25 %) from 0 to 15 days but E (400 mg) showed maximum reduction in average percentage LDL to 39.07 % from 0 to 15 day as compared to F (200 mg) and F. In contrary no satisfactory reduction was observed for rest of lipid profile as compare to standard (table: 5.25 and 5.26).

Table: 5.14: Effect of Polyherbal formulations on change in Blood glucose level and body weight from 0 day to 15th days (n =5)

Groups	No.	Dose	Fasting Blood Glucose Level (mg/dl)	After 3rd day of STZ injection (0 hr.) mg/dl	After 3 hr. (mg/dl)	Day 5th (mg/dl)	Day 10th (mg/dl)	Day 15th (mg/dl)	Fasting Body weight (gm)	After 3rd day of STZ injection (0 hr.)gm	After 3 hr. (gm)	Day 5th (gm)	Day 10th (gm)	Day 15th (gm)
Ist (control)	5	2ml/kg b.wt.	65 77 64 61 81	73 81 69 79 86	79 81 69 78 80	75 78 73 79 77	81 80 76 75 78	84 79 82 76 80	153.12 150.02 156.78 160.32 152.48	153.55 150.23 156.88 160.40 152.53	153.55 150.23 156.89 160.40 152.53	153.63 150.29 156.98 160.43 152.55	153.78 150.38 157.11 160.55 152.66	153.97 150.42 157.50 160.56 152.96
IInd Diabetic Control	5	60mg/kg b.wt.	75 62 68 66 70	308 320 284 325 300	308 321 284 325 302	328 345 298 331 334	342 358 321 349 348	356 373 338 364 366	152.26 156.82 151.66 169.75 159.60	151.98 156.68 151.54 169.68 159.52	151.99 156.67 151.52 169.62 159.21	150.62 150.42 150.28 169.20 159.21	149.92 149.82 149.95 169.01 159.00	149.84 149.83 149.64 168.70 158.82
IIIrd Std Glibenclamide	5	5mg/kg b.wt.	68 60 69 64 73	257 289 265 350 312	228 260 248 318 280	176 214 193 255 224	126 161 129 187 166	89 97 88 116 107	150.95 151.25 168.74 165.53 160.23	149.50 151.02 168.23 165.22 159.90	149.60 151.12 168.29 165.29 159.95	149.75 151.66 168.50 165.91 160.52	150.11 151.96 168.87 165.91 160.52	150.52 152.50 169.42 166.66 160.88
IVth F-A 200mg/kg g.b.wt	5	200 mg/kg b.wt.	69 88 82 75 80	262 280 314 299 276	251 269 298 283 261	220 231 250 226 225	186 185 196 190 180	160 134 150 143 132	170.05 165.75 155.52 150.04 156.01	169.98 165.82 155.02 150.01 155.92	169.98 165.83 155.02 150.01 155.92	170.02 165.85 155.43 150.34 155.95	170.28 165.91 155.50 150.38 155.97	170.31 165.93 155.54 150.41 155.99
Vth	5	400	72	295	282	236	187	142	168.35	168.09	168.09	168.14	168.16	168.26

Chapter 5 — Results and Observations

F-A 400 mg/kg b.wt			60	266	251	218	184	128	150.92	150.78	150.77	150.83	150.88	150.93
			62	307	292	254	214	148	151.72	151.57	151.57	151.67	151.54	151.83
			61	312	298	255	206	150	158.42	158.37	158.37	158.46	158.54	158.59
			65	272	259	221	178	131	160.14	160.10	160.10	160.15	160.27	160.38
VIth F-B 200 mg/kg	5	200 mg/kg b.wt.	66	378	356	298	234	144	186.65	185.50	185.52	185.71	185.94	186.12
			50	323	304	245	188	123	191.43	190.98	190.99	191.24	191.43	191.56
			63	350	327	268	205	133	178.66	177.82	177.86	177.92	178.10	178.33
			68	286	268	222	174	119	189.52	188.62	188.62	188.69	188.81	189.02
			72	272	255	206	157	104	193.21	192.50	192.51	192.58	192.63	192.78
VIIth F-B 400 mg/kg	5	400 mg/kg b.wt.	75	306	285	233	173	111	171.54	171.38	171.40	171.63	171.88	172.23
			79	256	235	189	141	89	183.23	183.03	183.06	183.29	183.35	183.57
			70	319	293	237	178	115	169.67	169.48	169.49	169.57	169.72	170.02
			66	328	309	250	191	119	175.89	175.71	175.71	175.93	176.12	176.28
			68	292	270	219	164	106	180.02	179.50	179.51	179.78	179.94	180.26
VIIIth F-C 200 mg/kg	5	200 mg/kg b.wt.	84	253	236	198	151	102	175.75	175.02	175.02	175.20	175.30	175.55
			62	289	270	224	173	116	192.45	192.23	192.24	192.30	192.38	192.42
			76	252	238	196	150	100	169.78	168.50	168.51	168.60	168.77	168.82
			65	291	272	225	174	117	176.92	175.23	175.24	175.29	175.41	175.55
			69	286	273	226	171	115	186.53	185.23	185.23	185.27	185.35	185.55
IXth F-C 400mg/kg b.wt	5	400 mg/kg b.wt.	76	290	277	231	182	131	170.42	169.82	169.83	169.96	170.10	170.22
			65	315	312	260	203	142	169.92	169.32	169.32	169.45	169.64	169.88
			79	303	289	241	191	137	187.45	187.02	187.03	187.24	187.38	187.52
			82	282	269	229	181	127	192.92	191.50	191.51	191.59	191.66	191.72
			69	288	272	231	187	130	190.52	190.00	190.00	190.18	190.24	190.35
Xth F-D 200 mg/kg	5	200 mg/kg	68	352	344	277	208	132	174.90	173.32	173.32	173.46	174.17	174.68
			73	341	318	260	205	109	165.96	165.04	165.34	165.59	165.74	165.87

200mg/kg b.wt		b.wt.	71	362	334	269	208	140	170.99	170.54	170.54	170.65	170.84	170.97
			66	302	281	228	182	122	169.45	168.76	168.76	168.90	169.20	169.42
			75	278	258	211	163	103	166.78	166.23	166.23	166.35	166.59	166.75
XIth F-D 400 mg/kg b.wt	5	400 mg/kg b.wt.	72	312	289	224	171	100	173.39	172.23	172.23	172.34	172.68	173.31
			69	268	247	193	143	97	164.21	163.65	163.65	163.78	163.97	163.35
			74	322	294	237	173	114	171.56	170.02	170.02	170.34	170.49	170.54
			68	331	310	247	179	111	159.75	158.78	158.79	158.94	159.23	159.69
			66	287	260	204	153	97	169.74	168.99	168.89	169.23	169.56	169.75
XIIth F-E 200 mg/kg b.wt	5	200 mg/kg b.wt.	74	283	275	212	148	80	164.35	164.37	164.32	164.46	164.89	165.01
			72	292	286	226	169	120	165.75	165.83	165.70	165.86	165.93	165.98
			68	312	301	267	201	130	171.08	170.38	170.25	170.63	170.74	170.82
			73	275	267	221	167	126	158.39	158.33	158.28	158.35	158.35	158.40
			69	296	288	216	171	124	163.09	162.64	162.45	162.72	163.02	163.11
XIIIth F-E 400 mg/kg b.wt	5	400 mg/kg b.wt.	66	268	257	223	187	80	168.35	168.09	168.09	168.14	168.16	168.26
			79	282	274	233	182	108	150.92	150.77	150.78	150.83	150.88	150.93
			75	309	301	256	192	125	151.72	151.57	151.57	151.67	151.78	151.83
			78	311	306	249	180	122	158.42	158.37	158.37	158.54	158.54	158.59
			63	289	271	237	178	113	160.14	160.10	160.10	160.15	160.27	160.38
XIVth F-F 200 mg/kg b.wt	5	200 mg/kg b.wt.	80	266	248	209	174	112	172.98	172.38	172.38	172.67	172.84	172.99
			66	284	268	225	170	110	167.86	167.43	167.43	167.63	165.74	165.84
			68	296	280	244	204	141	157.98	157.85	157.85	158.01	158.23	158.34
			72	288	264	228	185	130	168.34	168.01	168.01	168.26	168.30	168.35
			76	289	272	233	190	130	156.86	155.89	155.89	156.23	156.78	156.84
XVth F-F 400 mg/kg b.wt	5	400 mg/kg b.wt.	70	287	273	241	194	137	164.09	163.21	163.21	163.45	163.64	163.89
			68	320	312	265	211	152	171.23	171.03	171.01	171.32	171.78	171.82
			75	318	305	264	210	158	158.43	157.25	157.25	157.39	157.40	157.46
			80	294	278	243	197	149	163.76	163.48	163.48	163.69	163.73	163.78
			68	286	268	230	184	139	166.75	160.32	160.32	160.49	160.62	160.76

Results and Observations

Table 5.15: Effect of Polyherbal formulations on change in Fasting Blood glucose level in albino wistar rats 0 to 15 days (Mean ± S.D) n=5

Groups	Fasting Blood Glucose Level (mg/dl) after 18 hrs.	After 3rd day of STZ injection (0 hr./0 day) mg/dl	After 3 hr. (mg/dl)	Day 5th (mg/dl)	Day 10th (mg/dl)	Day 15th (mg/dl)
Normal Control	69.6±3.94	77.6±2.99	77.4±2.15	76.4±1.07	78.0±1.14	80.2±1.35
Diabetic Control	68.2±2.15	307.4±7.31	308±7.31	327.2±7.84	343.6±6.20	359.4±5.99
Standard Glibenclamide (5mg/kg)	66.8±2.22	294.6±16.87	266.8±15.33	212.4±13.51	153.8±11.59	99.4±5.37
Test F-A(200 mg/kg)	78.8±3.21	286.2±9.12	272.4±8.26	230.4±5.20	187.4±2.67	143.8±5.18
Test F-A(400mg/kg)	64.0±2.16	290.4±9.21	276.4±9.19	236.8±7.84	193.8±6.88	139.8±4.43
Test F-B(200 mg/kg)	63.8±3.74	321.8±19.64	302.0±18.58	247.8±16.35	191.6±13.22	124.6±6.72
Test F-B (400mg/kg)	71.6±2.37	300.2±12.61	278.4±12.54	225.6±10.40	169.4±8.33	108.0±2.74
Test F-C (200 mg/kg)	71.2±3.96	274.2±8.89	257.8±8.51	213.8±6.87	163.8±5.45	110.0±3.70
Test F-C (400mg/kg)	74.2±3.15	295.6±5.93	283.8±7.83	238.4±5.79	188.8±3.97	133.4±2.69
Test F-D(200 mg/kg)	70.6±1.63	327±15.92	307±16.27	249±12.62	193.2±8.98	121.2±6.89
Test F-D(400mg/kg)	69.8±1.42	304±11.62	280±11.54	221±10.03	163.8±6.77	103.8±3.62
Test F-E (200 mg/kg)	71.2±1.15	291.6±6.26	283.4±5.81	228.4±9.93	171.2±8.51	116±9.14
Test F-E (400mg/kg)	72.2±3.24	291.8±8.16	281.8±9.34	239.6±5.84	183.8±2.53	109.6±8.00
Test F-F (200 mg/kg)	72.4±2.56	284.6±5.03	266.4±5.30	227.8±5.70	184.6±5.91	124.6±5.91
Test F-F (400mg/kg)	72.2±2.33	301±7.48	287.2±8.90	248.6±6.86	199.2±5.09	147±3.96

P values < 0.0001 Values are Mean ± SE from 5 animals in each group.

Table 5.16: Total decrease in Percentage (%) of Average Blood glucose level from 0 day to 15 day for all six Poly herbal formulations

Treatment	Dose (mg/kg b.wt)	Average decrease in BGL from 0 day to 15th day	Observations
Standard (Glibenclamide)	5 mg/kg	66.2%	Showed maximum decrease in average BGL to 58.6 mg/dl between day 5th to day 10th
Formulation A	200 mg/kg	49.7%	Showed maximum decrease in average BGL to 43.4 mg/dl between day 10th to day 15th
	400 mg/kg	51.8%	Showed maximum decrease in average BGL to 54 mg/dl between day 10th to day 15th
Formulation B	200 mg/kg	61.2%	Showed maximum decrease in average BGL to 67 mg/dl between day 10th to day 15th
	400mg/kg	64.02%	Showed maximum reduction in average BGL to 61.4 mg/dl between day 10th to day 15th
Formulation C	200mg/kg	59.8%	Lower dose is most effective as compared to higher dose and it showed maximum reduction in average BGL to 68 mg/dl between day 5th to day 10th
	400mg/kg	54.8%	Higher dose is less effective and it showed maximum reduction in average BGL to 55.4 mg/dl between day 10th to day 15th
Formulation D	200 mg/kg	62.9%	Showed maximum decrease in average BGL to 72 mg/dl between day 10th to day 15th

	400 mg/kg	65.8%	**Showed maximum reduction in average BGL from 0th to 15th days as compared to other developed polyherbal combinations**
Formulation E	200 mg/kg	60.2%	Showed maximum decrease in average BGL to 57.2 mg/dl between day 5th to day 10th
	400mg/kg	62.4%	**Showed maximum reduction in average BGL to 74.2 mg/dl from day 10th to day 15th as compared to other polyherbal**
Formulation F	200mg/kg	56.2%	**Lower dose is most effective as compared to higher dose** and it showed maximum reduction in average BGL to 60 mg/dl between day 5th to day 10th
	400mg/kg	51.1%	Higher dose is less effective and it showed maximum reduction in average BGL to 52.2 mg/dl (26.20%) between day 10th to day 15th

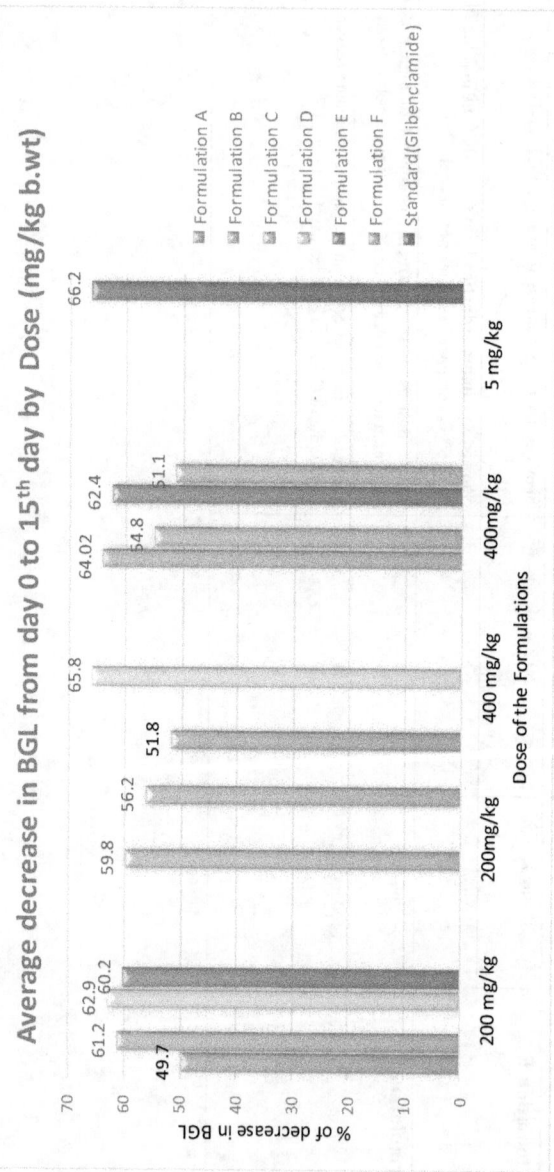

Figure 5.1 : Average decrease in percentage in Blood Glucose Level from 0 to 15th day

Table 5.17: Effect of Polyherbal formulation A (FA) on change in biochemical parameters of blood plasma in albino wistar rats from 0 day to 15th day

Parameters	Group I (Control)		Group II (Negative control)		Group III (Standard)		Group IV 200 mg		Group V 400 mg	
	0 day	After 15th day	0 day	After 15th day	0 day	After 15th day	0 day	After 15th day	0 day	After 15th day
Cholesterol	47.5	50.7	85.6	95.9	113.4	58.4	96.4	78.2	84.5	49.3
	48.7	49.0	91.6	112.6	96.7	48.3	120.4	91.3	93.9	58.6
	55.0	60.2	98.4	126.4	126.5	49.4	98.9	71.7	117.8	80.8
	50.3	48.1	88.2	102.4	109.4	46.7	104.4	79.4	111.9	72.9
	62.0	55.3	112.4	126.6	89.4	38.7	85.6	59.2	107.8	66.6
Triglycerides	59.8	61.7	166.0	212.9	155.2	71.2	125.3	79.5	115.7	64.5
	76.2	80.4	97.0	140.2	93.4	49.6	134.2	99.16	96.9	46.8
	60.4	60.9	113.8	143.8	133.4	73.5	128.7	93.1	129.5	77.8
	68.6	69.9	99.2	124.5	148.9	70.5	106.8	75.7	133.7	84.4
	68.4	67.6	84.3	111.7	138.6	67.3	112.4	78.8	118.9	64.6
SGOT	10.8	11.2	68.2	72.3	49.1	15.2	50.3	30.2	56.7	25.4
	25.2	26.7	59.5	74.6	63.2	20.2	47.6	18.3	45.2	20.0
	20.5	11.4	52.6	62.0	58.4	26.3	49.2	21.4	43.8	16.3
	31.6	30.2	49.0	60.1	41.8	13.1	60.4	39.2	58.4	18.4
	13.7	18.2	70.1	82.4	60.2	21.5	54.2	22.3	53.5	34.3
SGPT	24.6	26.3	62.4	71.2	68.3	17.2	71.9	20.1	75.2	26.2
	29.2	31.4	58.0	78.8	73.2	25.3	69.8	28.3	60.0	19.3
	30.1	32.6	59.5	69.2	69.6	21.3	59.2	31.2	63.4	20.1
	18.0	22.3	70.1	81.9	72.4	19.6	81.3	45.2	71.3	18.3
	15.6	18.7	68.0	85.6	68.6	20.4	90.0	48.2	78.6	21.3
Creatinine	0.48	0.52	1.54	1.72	1.59	0.92	1.61	1.33	1.77	1.53
	0.53	0.58	1.63	1.69	1.63	1.11	1.67	1.30	1.64	1.49
	0.61	0.63	1.62	1.82	1.57	0.72	1.73	1.52	1.58	1.24
	0.42	0.69	1.58	1.92	1.88	0.69	1.59	1.10	1.91	1.31
	1.12	1.15	1.42	1.78	1.92	1.23	1.79	1.58	1.62	0.62
Urea	30.2	31.2	86.7	91.2	75.2	23.2	69.3	38.4	78.3	41.2
	29.2	30.4	40.4	54.2	77.6	26.2	72.5	40.1	77.9	38.3

24.6	25.6	73.8	80.1	68.3	19.4	77.9	44.6	66.1	29.4
28.2	26.2	78.4	86.6	88.7	31.4	82.3	50.3	81.5	50.2
22.3	24.0	93.4	98.3	90.2	35.3	73.4	39.2	69.8	30.4
HDL									
40.1	35.0	21.2	15.2	30.0	40.0	17.6	21.0	18.4	26.4
35.8	40.3	20.2	12.0	20.1	41.3	21.3	29.4	23.7	29.0
34.4	41.7	18.9	10.0	18.6	35.3	24.6	30.4	21.0	29.4
35.3	38.5	19.9	12.2	15.2	36.2	20.0	28.6	39.4	45.0
41.0	36.2	30.2	18.1	20.2	38.1	19.2	24.6	28.3	36.4
LDL									
22.0	24.7	58.8	62.3	58.4	25.0	66.8	42.0	59.7	31.2
30.2	32.3	60.2	71.4	56.4	24.8	62.8	45.1	55.8	36.0
24.4	20.2	65.4	69.2	68.3	29.4	72.1	56.3	60.3	34.6
28.6	29.0	71.2	76.7	67.7	20.4	75.6	60.1	71.7	50.0
23.4	30.4	80.4	83.4	60.0	25.4	68.3	52.4	67.8	38.4

Results and Observations

Table 5.18: Effect of Polyherbal formulation B (FB) on change in biochemical parameters of blood plasma in albino wistar rats from 0 day to 15th day

Parameters	Group I (Control)		Group control) II (Negative		Group III (Standard)		Group IV 200 mg		Group V 400 mg	
	0 day	After 15th day	0 day	After 15th day	0 day	After 15th day	0 day	After 15th day	0 day	After 15th day
Cholesterol	47.5	50.7	85.6	95.9	113.4	58.4	133.8	91.5	91.0	58.4
	48.7	49.0	91.6	112.6	96.7	48.3	125.2	80.4	89.5	57.8
	55.0	60.2	98.4	126.4	126.5	49.4	110.8	65.7	108.6	77.7
	50.3	48.1	88.2	102.4	109.4	46.7	96.4	55.8	111.8	76.3
	62.0	55.3	112.4	126.6	89.4	38.7	106.5	58.4	125.5	92.1
Triglycerides	59.8	61.7	166.0	212.9	155.2	71.2	129.7	82.2	150.4	118.5
	76.2	80.4	97.0	140.2	93.4	49.6	162.1	115.4	132.4	99.1
	60.4	60.9	113.8	143.8	133.4	73.5	94.5	46.5	119.3	86.6
	68.6	69.9	99.2	124.5	148.9	70.5	134.1	90.4	97.0	66.2
	68.4	67.6	84.3	111.7	138.6	67.3	142.0	100.4	138.2	102.8
SGOT	10.8	11.2	68.2	72.3	49.1	15.2	58.2	26.1	65.4	41.1
	25.2	26.7	59.5	74.6	63.2	20.2	60.4	26.3	60.7	35.4
	20.5	11.4	52.6	62.0	58.4	26.3	56.7	17.8	77.8	54.0
	31.6	30.2	49.0	60.1	41.8	13.1	65.8	30.1	58.5	35.4
	13.7	18.2	70.1	82.4	60.2	21.5	68.9	32.1	64.5	37.7
SGPT	24.6	26.3	62.4	71.2	68.3	17.2	66.6	34.2	79.6	56.8
	29.2	31.4	58.0	78.8	73.2	25.3	60.4	20.9	57.4	32.8
	30.1	32.6	59.5	69.2	69.6	21.3	55.1	20.2	73.7	51.8
	18.0	22.3	70.1	81.9	72.4	19.6	72.5	39.1	67.8	42.7
	15.6	18.7	68.0	85.6	68.6	20.4	80.5	44.4	72.1	44.2

Creatinine	0.48	0.52	1.54	1.72	1.59	0.92	1.58	0.66	1.56	0.93
	0.53	0.58	1.63	1.69	1.63	1.11	1.68	0.83	1.68	1.01
	0.61	0.63	1.62	1.82	1.57	0.72	1.54	0.58	1.84	1.21
	0.42	0.69	1.58	1.92	1.88	0.69	1.89	1.05	1.62	0.89
	1.12	1.15	1.42	1.78	1.92	1.23	1.76	0.89	1.59	0.88
Urea	30.2	31.2	86.7	91.2	75.2	23.2	79.8	48.8	105.7	86.2
	29.2	30.4	40.4	54.2	77.6	26.2	64.7	35.2	74.9	58.7
	24.6	25.6	73.8	80.1	68.3	19.4	111.8	87.2	102.4	87.5
	28.2	26.2	78.4	86.6	88.7	31.4	92.4	69.2	90.0	73.7
	22.3	24.0	93.4	98.3	90.2	35.3	89.6	64.7	100.8	83.4
HDL	40.1	35.0	21.2	15.2	30.0	40.0	15.9	29.7	22.7	32.5
	35.8	40.3	20.2	12.0	20.1	41.3	20.8	36.7	20.1	28.8
	34.4	41.7	18.9	10.0	18.6	35.3	10.8	27.2	18.4	27.6
	35.3	38.5	19.9	12.2	15.2	36.2	24.2	36.5	15.7	25.3
	41.0	36.2	30.2	18.1	20.2	38.1	18.7	34.4	23.8	30.7
LDL	22.0	24.7	58.8	62.3	58.4	25.0	78.5	56.2	63.7	52.6
	30.2	32.3	60.2	71.4	56.4	24.8	66.7	46.9	80.8	68.4
	24.4	20.2	65.4	69.2	68.3	29.4	58.3	37.8	69.5	61.7
	28.6	29.0	71.2	76.7	67.7	20.4	64.2	41.6	78.5	68.9
	23.4	30.4	80.4	83.4	60.0	25.4	80.0	55.3	84.7	76.2

Results and Observations

Table 5.19: Effect of Polyherbal formulation C (FC) on change in biochemical parameters of blood plasma in albino wistar rats from 0 day to 15th day

Parameters	Group I (Control)		Group II (Negative control)		Group III (Standard)		Group IV 200 mg		Group V 400 mg	
	0 day	After 15th day	0 day	After 15th day	0 day	After 15th day	0 day	After 15th day	0 day	After 15th day
Cholesterol	47.5	50.7	85.6	95.9	113.4	58.4	120.1	90.1	113.3	80.4
	48.7	49.0	91.6	112.6	96.7	48.3	115.6	88.7	125.0	102.1
	55.0	60.2	98.4	126.4	126.5	49.4	98.9	82.3	110.4	88.0
	50.3	48.1	88.2	102.4	109.4	46.7	107.3	89.4	91.3	78.4
	62.0	55.3	112.4	126.6	89.4	38.7	128.8	111.4	85.4	71.2
Triglycerides	59.8	61.7	166.0	212.9	155.2	71.2	163.3	135.8	165.3	142.3
	76.2	80.4	97.0	140.2	93.4	49.6	154.7	129.4	134.8	120.1
	60.4	60.9	113.8	143.8	133.4	73.5	120.4	101.5	150.3	121.3
	68.6	69.9	99.2	124.5	148.9	70.5	138.6	116.2	112.6	96.4
	68.4	67.6	84.3	111.7	138.6	67.3	126.6	115.3	96.8	79.8
SGOT	10.8	11.2	68.2	72.3	49.1	15.2	50.7	31.2	45.9	28.2
	25.2	26.7	59.5	74.6	63.2	20.2	54.2	36.0	48.6	30.1
	20.5	11.4	52.6	62.0	58.4	26.3	62.3	46.8	69.5	51.2
	31.6	30.2	49.0	60.1	41.8	13.1	48.1	24.3	75.6	63.2
	13.7	18.2	70.1	82.4	60.2	21.5	94.0	70.1	80.2	75.3
SGPT	24.6	26.3	62.4	71.2	68.3	17.2	94.1	82.0	78.2	61.7
	29.2	31.4	58.0	78.8	73.2	25.3	91.7	85.1	85.8	67.8
	30.1	32.6	59.5	69.2	69.6	21.3	68.8	49.2	82.1	66.8
	18.0	22.3	70.1	81.9	72.4	19.6	90.0	75.4	93.0	75.5
	15.6	18.7	68.0	85.6	68.6	20.4	112.2	96.2	101.2	82.3
Creatinine	0.48	0.52	1.54	1.72	1.59	0.92	1.52	0.89	1.71	1.48
	0.53	0.58	1.63	1.69	1.63	1.11	1.63	0.72	1.68	1.55
	0.61	0.63	1.62	1.82	1.57	0.72	1.58	0.92	1.59	1.49
	0.42	0.69	1.58	1.92	1.88	0.69	1.53	0.98	1.62	0.91
	1.12	1.15	1.42	1.78	1.92	1.23	1.64	1.12	1.51	0.82

Urea										
	30.2	31.2	86.7	91.2	75.2	23.2	174.7	96.5	51.3	39.2
	29.2	30.4	40.4	54.2	77.6	26.2	101.6	46.5	62.8	48.7
	24.6	25.6	73.8	80.1	68.3	19.4	162.4	90.4	74.8	61.4
	28.2	26.2	78.4	86.6	88.7	31.4	126.5	84.7	80.3	67.9
	22.3	24.0	93.4	98.3	90.2	35.3	135.4	102.1	59.8	46.6
HDL										
	40.1	35.0	21.2	15.2	30.0	40.0	16.8	20.0	11.2	22.2
	35.8	40.3	20.2	12.0	20.1	41.3	19.6	25.1	14.6	26.4
	34.4	41.7	18.9	10.0	18.6	35.3	28.0	30.2	19.6	29.3
	35.3	38.5	19.9	12.2	15.2	36.2	26.7	32.1	20.3	32.4
	41.0	36.2	30.2	18.1	20.2	38.1	17.9	25.0	16.4	30.2
LDL										
	22.0	24.7	58.8	62.3	58.4	25.0	81.5	70.4	92.1	75.0
	30.2	32.3	60.2	71.4	56.4	24.8	69.3	31.2	103.2	91.2
	24.4	20.2	65.4	69.2	68.3	29.4	86.0	65.2	100.4	86.3
	28.6	29.0	71.2	76.7	67.7	20.4	78.3	69.0	88.3	74.3
	23.4	30.4	80.4	83.4	60.0	25.4	77.2	70.1	90.4	70.0

Table 5.20: Effect of Polyherbal formulation D (FD) on change in biochemical parameters of blood plasma in albino wistar rats from 0 day to 15th day

Parameters	Group I (Control)		Group II (Negative control)		Group III (Standard)		Group IV 200 mg		Group V 400 mg	
	0 day	After 15th day	0 day	After 15th day	0 day	After 15th day	0 day	After 15th day	0 day	After 15th day
Cholesterol	47.5	50.7	85.6	95.9	113.4	58.4	136.4	84.6	125.6	61.8
	48.7	49.0	91.6	112.6	96.7	48.3	162.1	94.1	151.4	82.6
	55.0	60.2	98.4	126.4	126.5	49.4	158.3	71.5	168.6	90.4
	50.3	48.1	88.2	102.4	109.4	46.7	129.8	65.6	158.6	106.5
	62.0	55.3	112.4	126.6	89.4	38.7	164.3	96.3	182.6	77.9
Triglycerides	59.8	61.7	166.0	212.9	155.2	71.2	150.6	83.6	138.2	70.5
	76.2	80.4	97.0	140.2	93.4	49.6	139.8	68.4	167.5	81.4
	60.4	60.9	113.8	143.8	133.4	73.5	149.6	70.1	156.4	79.4
	68.6	69.9	99.2	124.5	148.9	70.5	126.7	66.7	129.5	69.3
	68.4	67.6	84.3	111.7	138.6	67.3	161.9	90.4	96.8	54.7
SGOT	10.8	11.2	68.2	72.3	49.1	15.2	78.9	30.4	79.5	29.5
	25.2	26.7	59.5	74.6	63.2	20.2	80.1	29.5	84.6	33.6
	20.5	11.4	52.6	62.0	58.4	26.3	63.4	26.5	95.4	51.7
	31.6	30.2	49.0	60.1	41.8	13.1	66.6	37.1	75.8	26.5
	13.7	18.2	70.1	82.4	60.2	21.5	91.4	41.3	88.1	46.5
SGPT	24.6	26.3	62.4	71.2	68.3	17.2	86.4	30.8	67.9	27.9
	29.2	31.4	58.0	78.8	73.2	25.3	73.6	36.4	79.9	37.2
	30.1	32.6	59.5	69.2	69.6	21.3	68.7	41.5	76.3	31.6
	18.0	22.3	70.1	81.9	72.4	19.6	69.6	42.7	76.8	21.2
	15.6	18.7	68.0	85.6	68.6	20.4	82.7	44.4	63.8	28.6
Creatinine	0.48	0.52	1.54	1.72	1.59	0.92	1.71	0.90	1.68	0.44
	0.53	0.58	1.63	1.69	1.63	1.11	1.67	0.84	1.85	0.68
	0.61	0.63	1.62	1.82	1.57	0.72	1.59	1.12	1.63	0.84
	0.42	0.69	1.58	1.92	1.88	0.69	1.84	0.67	1.56	0.89

	1.12	1.15	1.42	1.78	1.92	1.23	1.36	0.70	1.34	0.57
Urea	30.2	31.2	86.7	91.2	75.2	23.2	96.4	71.3	111.7	81.2
	29.2	30.4	40.4	54.2	77.6	26.2	108.6	80.1	128.9	86.3
	24.6	25.6	73.8	80.1	68.3	19.4	123.7	83.6	139.4	112.3
	28.2	26.2	78.4	86.6	88.7	31.4	152.6	122.4	161.4	123.8
	22.3	24.0	93.4	98.3	90.2	35.3	161.7	138.4	170.2	140.1
HDL	40.1	35.0	21.2	15.2	30.0	40.0	15.8	30.2	11.3	35.7
	35.8	40.3	20.2	12.0	20.1	41.3	21.3	40.8	16.3	38.2
	34.4	41.7	18.9	10.0	18.6	35.3	28.2	45.4	20.1	34.3
	35.3	38.5	19.9	12.2	15.2	36.2	18.6	34.2	18.4	40.1
	41.0	36.2	30.2	18.1	20.2	38.1	13.6	29.1	10.0	29.2
LDL	22.0	24.7	58.8	62.3	58.4	25.0	78.6	56.4	66.7	50.1
	30.2	32.3	60.2	71.4	56.4	24.8	68.1	47.3	80.4	72.3
	24.4	20.2	65.4	69.2	68.3	29.4	83.4	58.4	69.6	59.4
	28.6	29.0	71.2	76.7	67.7	20.4	68.9	43.1	78.3	64.4
	23.4	30.4	80.4	83.4	60.0	25.4	70.1	58.2	83.6	70.2

Chapter 5 Results and Observations

Table 5.21: Effect of Polyherbal formulation E (FE) on Change in biochemical parameters of blood plasma in albino wistar rats from 0 day to 15th day

Parameters	Group I (Control)		Group II (Negative control)		Group III (Standard)		Group IV 200 mg		Group V 400 mg	
	0 day	After 15th day	0 day	After 15th day	0 day	After 15th day	0 day	After 15th day	0 day	After 15th day
Cholesterol	47.5	50.7	85.6	95.9	113.4	58.4	146.6	84.2	98.6	50.4
	48.7	49.0	91.6	112.6	96.7	48.3	139.5	111.3	141.2	81.6
	55.0	60.2	98.4	126.4	126.5	49.4	129.6	100.2	133.6	100.4
	50.3	48.1	88.2	102.4	109.4	46.7	116.7	94.3	119.8	86.5
	62.0	55.3	112.4	126.6	89.4	38.7	138.7	121.3	127.3	79.5
Triglycerides	59.8	61.7	166.0	212.9	155.2	71.2	148.9	120.4	176.2	142.3
	76.2	80.4	97.0	140.2	93.4	49.6	171.3	138.6	153.6	139.6
	60.4	60.9	113.8	143.8	133.4	73.5	182.7	154.1	139.2	90.6
	68.6	69.9	99.2	124.5	148.9	70.5	159.1	116.2	154.3	130.2
	68.4	67.6	84.3	111.7	138.6	67.3	166.6	135.2	129.1	91.6
SGOT	10.8	11.2	68.2	72.3	49.1	15.2	56.4	33.6	55.9	31.2
	25.2	26.7	59.5	74.6	63.2	20.2	67.3	39.4	58.7	30.2
	20.5	11.4	52.6	62.0	58.4	26.3	58.7	30.4	68.9	47.3
	31.6	30.2	49.0	60.1	41.8	13.1	72.4	42.5	75.3	61.2
	13.7	18.2	70.1	82.4	60.2	21.5	62.6	45.6	81.3	66.2
SGPT	24.6	26.3	62.4	71.2	68.3	17.2	97.4	80.6	77.8	51.3
	29.2	31.4	58.0	78.8	73.2	25.3	94.2	85.3	86.2	66.8
	30.1	32.6	59.5	69.2	69.6	21.3	82.4	61.4	89.3	63.7
	18.0	22.3	70.1	81.9	72.4	19.6	90.0	70.3	90.4	75.3
	15.6	18.7	68.0	85.6	68.6	20.4	113.5	89.2	112.3	88.3
Creatinine	0.48	0.52	1.54	1.72	1.59	0.92	1.68	1.29	1.76	1.48
	0.53	0.58	1.63	1.69	1.63	1.11	1.53	1.19	1.71	1.41
	0.61	0.63	1.62	1.82	1.57	0.72	1.58	1.13	1.53	1.21

	0.42	0.69	1.58	1.92	1.88	0.69	1.72	1.61	1.94	1.35
	1.12	1.15	1.42	1.78	1.92	1.23	1.60	1.42	1.63	0.92
Urea	30.2	31.2	86.7	91.2	75.2	23.2	98.4	36.5	119.1	41.5
	29.2	30.4	40.4	54.2	77.6	26.2	113.4	48.1	99.1	40.2
	24.6	25.6	73.8	80.1	68.3	19.4	86.5	50.1	134.1	112.1
	28.2	26.2	78.4	86.6	88.7	31.4	79.6	41.2	136.4	106.7
	22.3	24.0	93.4	98.3	90.2	35.3	87.4	32.3	111.3	90.4
HDL	40.1	35.0	21.2	15.2	30.0	40.0	17.7	28.0	18.9	27.1
	35.8	40.3	20.2	12.0	20.1	41.3	23.8	32.6	22.7	34.3
	34.4	41.7	18.9	10.0	18.6	35.3	30.1	41.7	19.3	24.6
	35.3	38.5	19.9	12.2	15.2	36.2	22.6	37.6	25.4	36.4
	41.0	36.2	30.2	18.1	20.2	38.1	16.8	28.6	15.4	32.3
LDL	22.0	24.7	58.8	62.3	58.4	25.0	58.7	26.4	59.2	36.2
	30.2	32.3	60.2	71.4	56.4	24.8	66.4	29.7	52.3	30.1
	24.4	20.2	65.4	69.2	68.3	29.4	73.1	58.3	68.7	39.6
	28.6	29.0	71.2	76.7	67.7	20.4	69.1	51.3	73.4	52.3
	23.4	30.4	80.4	83.4	60.0	25.4	74.3	61.1	64.5	35.6

Table 5.22 : Effect of Polyherbal formulation F (FF) on Change in biochemical parameters of blood plasma in albino wistar rats from 0 day to 15th day n=5

Parameters	Group I (Control)		Group II (Negative control)		Group III (Standard)		Group IV 200 mg		Group V 400 mg	
	0 day	After 15th day	0 day	After 15th day	0 day	After 15th day	0 day	After 15th day	0 day	After 15th day
Cholesterol	47.5	50.7	85.6	95.9	113.4	58.4	141.1	89.3	132.6	128.1
	48.7	49.0	91.6	112.6	96.7	48.3	128.6	112.3	117.8	96.7
	55.0	60.2	98.4	126.4	126.5	49.4	113.4	92.4	121.3	100.2
	50.3	48.1	88.2	102.4	109.4	46.7	126.7	102.8	95.8	76.3
	62.0	55.3	112.4	126.6	89.4	38.7	138.5	122.6	129.1	108.6
Triglycerides	59.8	61.7	166.0	212.9	155.2	71.2	167.2	131.1	131.4	119.2
	76.2	80.4	97.0	140.2	93.4	49.6	155.7	120.2	129.7	101.6
	60.4	60.9	113.8	143.8	133.4	73.5	163.2	121.2	168.9	143.3
	68.6	69.9	99.2	124.5	148.9	70.5	138.1	117.6	159.2	121.6
	68.4	67.6	84.3	111.7	138.6	67.3	142.3	120.1	141.4	109.6
SGOT	10.8	11.2	68.2	72.3	49.1	15.2	57.8	36.1	49.6	28.2
	25.2	26.7	59.5	74.6	63.2	20.2	56.2	31.6	68.9	53.5
	20.5	11.4	52.6	62.0	58.4	26.3	63.6	48.9	72.3	60.1
	31.6	30.2	49.0	60.1	41.8	13.1	49.8	25.7	81.4	72.4
	13.7	18.2	70.1	82.4	60.2	21.5	95.6	74.1	82.6	75.6
SGPT	24.6	26.3	62.4	71.2	68.3	17.2	102.6	90.5	96.6	81.2
	29.2	31.4	58.0	78.8	73.2	25.3	69.8	51.2	98.9	85.4
	30.1	32.6	59.5	69.2	69.6	21.3	82.6	71.3	72.3	64.8
	18.0	22.3	70.1	81.9	72.4	19.6	96.3	80.6	115.8	102.4
	15.6	18.7	68.0	85.6	68.6	20.4	114.3	92.3	109.8	80.8

Creatinine	0.48	0.52	1.54	1.72	1.59	0.92	1.51	1.12	1.71	1.48
	0.53	0.58	1.63	1.69	1.63	1.11	1.62	1.14	1.62	1.15
	0.61	0.63	1.62	1.82	1.57	0.72	1.58	0.98	1.58	0.83
	0.42	0.69	1.58	1.92	1.88	0.69	1.68	1.25	0.98	0.61
	1.12	1.15	1.42	1.78	1.92	1.23	1.49	0.98	0.95	0.66
Urea	30.2	31.2	86.7	91.2	75.2	23.2	98.6	49.8	162.7	94.8
	29.2	30.4	40.4	54.2	77.6	26.2	96.8	52.1	129.8	112.1
	24.6	25.6	73.8	80.1	68.3	19.4	129.7	82.7	139.6	121.3
	28.2	26.2	78.4	86.6	88.7	31.4	139.6	112.8	172.4	98.9
	22.3	24.0	93.4	98.3	90.2	35.3	159.2	121.0	157.3	101.2
HDL	40.1	35.0	21.2	15.2	30.0	40.0	12.6	20.3	18.6	26.4
	35.8	40.3	20.2	12.0	20.1	41.3	15.9	34.2	17.9	29.3
	34.4	41.7	18.9	10.0	18.6	35.3	19.8	37.1	25.4	34.2
	35.3	38.5	19.9	12.2	15.2	36.2	18.1	32.0	19.4	28.4
	41.0	36.2	30.2	18.1	20.2	38.1	20.3	34.2	16.4	29.6
LDL	22.0	24.7	58.8	62.3	58.4	25.0	86.3	70.1	92.6	75.6
	30.2	32.3	60.2	71.4	56.4	24.8	78.6	68.6	106.4	92.3
	24.4	20.2	65.4	69.2	68.3	29.4	104.4	93.4	112.4	86.3
	28.6	29.0	71.2	76.7	67.7	20.4	88.6	74.3	89.8	73.4
	23.4	30.4	80.4	83.4	60.0	25.4	79.6	63.4	90.5	70.1

Table: 5.23: Effect of Formulations on Biochemical Parameters of blood plasma. Values are showed in mean ± SE from 5 animals in each group

Parameters	Normal Control		Diabetic Control		Standard Glibenclamide		Test A 200 mg		Test A 400 mg		Test B 200 mg		Test B 400 mg		Test C 200 mg		Test C 400 mg	
	0 Day	After 15 Day	0 Day	After 15 Day	0 Day	After 15 Day	0 Day	After 15 Day	0 Day	After 15 Day	0 day	After 15 day	0 Day	After 15 Day	0 Day	After 15 Day	0 Day	After 15 Day
Cholesterol	52.7±2.65	52.66±2.25	95.24±4.79	112.78±6.20	107.08±6.49	48.3±3.14	101.4±5.70	75.96±5.24	103.8±6.10	65.64±5.47	114.54±6.67	70.36±6.79	105.28±6.76	72.46±6.48	114.14±5.15	92.38±4.95	105.08±7.31	84.02±5.25
Triglycerides	66.68±3.03	68.1±3.51	112.06±14.27	146.62±17.53	133.9±10.81	66.42±4.32	121.48±5.13	85.25±4.57	118.94±6.42	67.62±6.47	132.48±1.00	86.98±11.53	127.46±9.11	94.64±8.74	140.72±8.13	119.64±5.98	131.96±2.38	111.98±1.84
SGOT	20.36±3.77	19.54±3.88	59.88±4.15	70.28±4.13	54.54±3.96	19.26±2.34	52.34±2.29	26.28±3.77	51.52±2.98	22.88±3.22	62.0±2.31	26.48±2.45	65.38±3.34	40.72±3.48	61.86±8.38	41.68±7.99	63.96±7.04	49.6±9.18
SGPT	23.5±2.91	26.26±2.64	63.6±2.35	77.34±3.12	70.42±1.00	20.76±1.32	74.4±5.24	34.6±5.28	69.7±3.50	21.04±1.38	67.02±4.46	31.76±4.85	70.12±3.69	45.66±4.11	91.36±6.90	77.58±7.85	88.06±4.09	70.82±3.62
Creatinine (mg/dl)	0.63±0.12	0.71±0.11	1.55±0.03	1.78±0.04	1.71±0.07	0.93±0.10	1.67±0.03	1.36±0.08	1.70±0.06	1.23±0.16	1.69±0.06	0.802±0.08	1.658±0.04	0.984±0.06	1.58±0.02	0.926±0.06	1.622±0.03	1.25±0.15

Chapter 5 — Results and Observations

Urea(mg/dl)	26.9±1.48	27.48±1.40	74.54±9.17	82.08±7.57	80.0±4.15	27.1±2.83	75.08±2.26	42.52±2.22	74.72±2.89	37.9±3.81	87.66±7.73	61.02±8.89	94.76±5.61	77.9±5.37	140.12±13.0	84.04±9.82	65.8±5.2	52.76±5.20
HDL (mg/dl)	37.32±1.34	38.34±1.24	22.08±2.06	13.5±1.41	20.82±2.46	38.18±1.12	20.54±1.17	26.8±1.75	26.16±3.69	33.24±3.37	18.08±2.26	32.9±1.90	20.14±1.46	28.98±1.24	21.8±2.31	26.48±2.13	16.42±1.66	28.1±1.76
LDL (mg/dl)	25.72±1.57	27.32±2.17	67.2±3.95	72.6±3.55	62.16±2.45	25.00±1.42	69.12±2.20	51.18±3.38	63.06±2.90	38.04±3.20	69.54±4.19	47.56±3.64	75.44±3.85	65.56±3.97	78.46±2.75	61.18±7.55	94.88±2.92	79.36±4.00

P values: <0.0001 significantly different from Control, Diabetic control

Table: 5.24: Effect of Formulations on Biochemical Parameters of blood. Values are mean ± SE from 5 animals in each group

Parameters	Normal Control		Diabetic Control		Standard Glibenclamide		Test D 200 mg		Test D 400 mg		Test E 200 mg		Test E 400 mg		Test F 200 mg		Test F 400 mg	
	0 Day	After 15 Day	0 Day	After 15 Day	0 Day	After 15 Day	0 Day	After 15 Day	0 Day	After 15 Day	0 day	After 15 day	0 Day	After 15 Day	0 Day	After 15 Day	0 Day	After 15 Day
Cholesterol	52.7 ±2.65	52.6 ±2.25	95.24 ±4.79	112.78 ±6.20	107.08 ±6.49	48.3 ±3.14	150.18 ±7.11	82.42 ±6.06	157.36 ±9.51	83.84 ±7.34	134.22 ±5.14	102.26 ±6.47	124.1 ±7.28	79.68 ±8.17	129.66 ±4.91	103.88 ±6.19	119.32 ±6.44	101.98 ±8.41
Triglycerides	66.68 ±3.03	68.1 ±3.51	112.06 ±14.27	146.62 ±17.53	133.9 ±10.81	66.42 ±4.32	137.68 ±12.20	71.06 ±4.73	145.72 ±5.90	75.84 ±4.71	165.72 ±5.68	132.9 ±6.79	150.48 ±7.96	118.86 ±11.51	153.3 ±5.69	122.04 ±2.34	146.12 ±7.74	119.06 ±7.02
SGOT	20.36 ±3.77	19.54 ±3.88	59.88 ±4.15	70.28 ±4.13	54.54 ±3.96	19.26 ±2.34	76.08 ±5.04	32.96 ±2.71	84.68 ±3.40	37.56 ±4.91	63.48 ±2.89	38.3 ±2.79	68.02 ±4.81	47.22 ±7.42	64.6± 8.05	43.28 ±8.59	70.96 ±5.94	57.96 ±8.54
SGPT	23.5 ±2.91	26.26 ±2.64	63.6 ±2.35	77.34 ±3.12	70.42 ±1.00	20.76 ±1.32	76.20 ±3.55	39.16 ±2.47	72.94 ±3.02	29.30 ±2.60	95.5 ±5.15	77.36 ±5.09	91.2 ±5.71	69.08 ±6.15	95.5 ±5.15	77.36 ±5.09	91.2 ±5.71	69.08 ±6.15

Creatinine (mg/dl)	0.63 ±0.12	0.71 ±0.11	1.55 ±0.03	1.78 ±0.04	1.71 ±0.07	0.93 ±0.10	1.63 ±0.07	0.84 ±0.08	1.61 ±0.08	0.68 ±0.08	1.62 ±0.03	1.32 ±0.08	1.71 ±0.06	1.27 ±0.09	1.62 ±0.03	1.32 ±0.08	1.71 ±0.06	1.27 ±0.09
Urea (mg/dl)	26.9 ±1.48	27.48 ±1.40	74.54 ±9.17	82.08 ±7.57	80.0 ±4.15	27.1 ±2.83	142.32 ±10.64	108.74 ±11.11	128.60 ±12.51	99.16 ±13.15	93.06 ±5.90	41.64 ±3.37	120 ±7.00	78.18 ±15.65	93.06 ±5.90	41.64 ±3.37	120.0 ±7.00	78.18 ±15.65
HDL (mg/dl)	37.32 ±1.34	38.34 ±1.24	22.08 ±2.06	13.5 ±1.41	20.82 ±2.46	38.18 ±1.12	19.50 ±2.53	35.94 ±3.12	15.22 ±1.97	35.50 ±1.86	22.2 ±2.39	33.7 ±2.63	20.34 ±1.71	30.94 ±2.21	22.2 ±2.39	33.7 ±2.63	20.34 ±1.71	30.94 ±2.21
LDL (mg/dl)	25.72 ±1.57	27.32 ±2.17	67.2 ±3.95	72.6 ±3.55	62.16 ±2.45	25.00 ±1.42	73.82 ±3.04	52.68 ±3.14	75.72 ±3.23	63.28 ±3.99	68.32 ±2.78	45.36 ±7.26	63.62 ±3.67	38.76 ±3.71	68.32 ±2.78	45.36 ±7.26	63.62 ±3.67	38.76 ±3.71

P values: <0.0001 significantly different from Control, Diabetic control

Table: 5.25: Average Percentage decreases in Biochemical parameters of blood serum of diabetic rats from 0 to 15th days for all the six Formulations

Treatment	Dose	Cholesterol	Triglycerides(TG)	SGOT	SGPT	Creatinine	Urea	HDL	LDL
Glibenclamide	5mg/kg	54.8%	50.3%	64.6%	70.5%	45.6%	66.1%	45.4%	59.7%
F-A	200 mg/kg	24.8%	29.8%	49.7%	53.5%	18.56%	43.3%	23.3%	25.9%
	400mg/kg	36.7%	43.1%	55.5%	69.8%	27.6%	49.2%	27.3%	39.6%
F-B	200 mg/kg	38.5%	34.3%	57.2%	52.5%	52.5%	30.3%	45.0%	31.6%
	400 mg/kg	31.1%	25.7%	37.7%	34.8%	40.6%	17.7%	30.5%	13.0%
F-C	200 mg/kg	19.0%	14.9%	32.6%	15.0%	41.3%	40.0%	17.6%	22.0%
	400 mg/kg	20.0%	15.1%	22.4%	19.5%	22.9%	19.8%	41.5%	16.3%
F-D	200 mg/kg	41.1%	37.96%	56.67%	48.60%	48.16%	22.89%	45.7%	28.70%
	400mg/kg	46.7%	48.38%	55.60%	59.83%	57.46%	23.59%	57.12%	16.42%
F-E	200 mg/kg	23.81%	19.80%	39.66%	18.99%	18.1%	55.25%	34.12%	33.60%
	400 mg/kg	35.79%	21.01%	30.57%	24.25%	25.7%	34.85%	34.25%	39.07%
F-F	200 mg/kg	19.88%	20.39%	33.01%	23.56%	30.30%	32.98%	45.05%	15.47%
	400 mg/kg	14.53%	18.51%	18.32%	15.97%	30.84%	30.65%	33.94%	19.11%

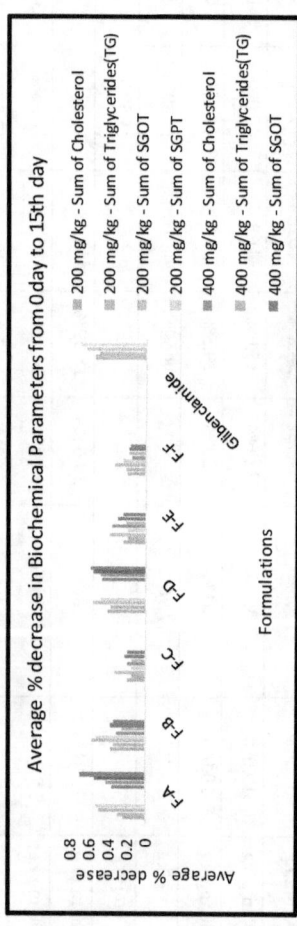

Figure 5.2: Average % decrease in biochemical parameters from 0 to 15th day

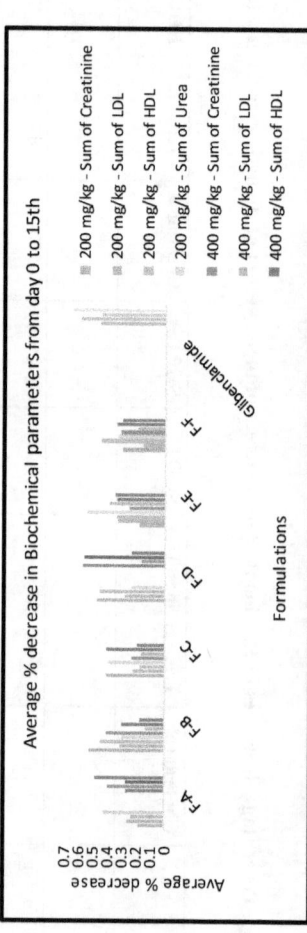

Figure 5.3: Average % decrease in biochemical parameters from 0 to 15th day

Table: 5.26: Analysis of other Biochemical Parameters

Treatment	Dose	Biochemical parameter maximum decreased from day 0th to day 15th	% decrease	Remarks
F-A	400 mg/kg b.wt.	SGPT, LDL	69.8%, 39.6	Decrease in SGPT is near to standard
F-B	200 mg/kg b.wt.	SGOT	57.2%	----
F-D	400 mg/kg b.wt.	TC, TG, Creatinine	46.7%, 48.3%, 57.46%	Decrease in Creatinine level is greater than Std.
F-E	200 mg/kg b.wt.	Urea	55.25%	-----

5.8 Quality control/Standardization of Polyherbal formulations

Some quality control parameters for polyherbal formulations were established and results are summarized as follows:

5.8.1 HPTLC fingerprinting

HPTLC fingerprinting showed the effective separation at 366 nm and 254 nm as shown in figure 5.40 to 5.46 and the R_f values with peak areas are shown in Chromatogram (At 254 nm: figure: 5.1 to figure: 5.20 and at 366 nm: figure:5.21 to figure:5.39)

- At 366 nm F-A showed 9 spots at R_f 0.14,0.27,0.34,0.40,0.44,0.49,0.53,0.56,0.96. In these R_f 0.14 corresponds to standard Piperine, R_f 0.56 corresponds to Standard Stigmasterol. At 254 nm the chromatogram of F-A showed 7 peaks with R_f (0.03, 0.04, 0.15, 0.24, 0.29, 0.38 and 0.46), R_f value 0.04 and 0.15 corresponds to standard Gallic acid and Piperine.

- For F-B, the HPTLC profiling showed 5 peaks with R_f (0.04, 0.16, 0.26, 0.40 and 0.49) in the chromatogram at 254 nm, band with R_f value 0.04 corresponds to standard Gallic acid and R_f 0.16 corresponds to Quercetin whereas at 366 nm chromatogram also showed 5 spots with R_f (0.08, 0.17, 0.40, 0.49, 0.56). R_f 0.56 corresponds to standard Stigmasterol and R_f 0.08 corresponds to standard Ellagic acid, Rutin.

- F-C: Chromatogram at 254 nm showed 7 peaks (R_f 0.03,0.15,0.23,0.27,0.56,0.68), band with R_f 0.15 corresponds to standard Piperine and 0.56 corresponds to standard Stigma sterol whereas at 366 nm it showed 3 peaks with R_f 0.13,0.25,0.48.

- F-D: Under 254 nm it showed 4 peaks with R_f value at 0.04, 0.22, 0.27, and 0.50 in which R_f value 0.04 and 0.50 corresponds to standard Gallic acid and Stigmasterol; under 366 nm it showed 5 peaks with R_f values at 0.11, 0.15, 0.24, 0.42 and 0.48. R_f value 0.15 corresponds to the standard compound Piperine.

- F-E: On analyzing under densitometer at 366 nm, the chromatogram of polyherbal mixture E showed 3 peaks while at 254 nm the chromatogram showed 9 peaks. Band with R_f value 0.14 corresponds to standard Piperine confirmed the presence of *Piper longum* while R_f 0.06,0.04 and 0.15 corresponds to standard Catechin and standard Gallic acid and Piperine.

- The chromatogram of polyherbal mixture F showed the presence of 9 peaks at 254nm while at 366 nm chromatogram showed 6peaks. R_f value 0.55, 0.05 corresponds to standard Stigmasterol, Gallic acid and 0.15 corresponds to Piperine.

Derivatization Results
- Results of HPTLC profiling after Derivatization of Polyherbals at 420 nm are shown in Chromatogram from page (figure:5.47 to figure 5.66)
- F-A showed the presence of 6 spots and R_f 0.64 and 0.73 corresponds to standard Catechin and Gallic acid.
- F-B chromatogram at 420 nm showed the presence of 7 peaks; band with R_f 0.03, 0.65 corresponds to Quercetin, Catechin.
- F-C showed the presence of 5 spots, R_f 0.03, 0.06 corresponds to standard Quercetin and Rutin.
- F-D chromatogram showed 4 spots and in this R_f 0.04 corresponds to Quercetin.
- F-E at 420 nm showed 3 peaks, band with 0.03 corresponds to standard Quercetin and R_f 0.92 corresponds to Piperine.
- F-F chromatogram at 420 nm showed 5 peaks, band with R_f 0.03, 0.66, 0.92 corresponds to Quercetin, Ellagic acid and Piperine.

Chapter 5 — Results and Observations

DESAGA ProQuant: Method for chromatogram

Name of Method:	Method for Chromatogram
Created by:	USER
Comment:	
Date/Time:	28-Nov-13 03:26:02 PM
Start coordinate X:	22.0 mm
Start coordinate Y:	12.0 mm
End coordinate Y:	135.0 mm
Number of lanes:	14
Distance of lanes:	12.0 [mm]
Mode:	Remission
Evaluation mode:	Extinction
Slit width:	4.00 mm
Slit height:	0.40 mm
Wavelength:	254 nm
Wavelength (Reference):	0 nm
Filter position:	Open
Signal:	positive
Lamp:	Deu/Tungsten
Maeander width:	0.0 mm
Subsoil correction for maeanderscan:	no
Resolution at measurement:	0.100 mm
Number of measurements/point:	1
Smoothing value:	None
Lane optimization:	no
Automatic zeroing:	yes
Signal range of graphic:	-1000 to 1000
Autom. evaluation after measurement:	yes
Window width:	2.00 mm
Threshold for peak detection:	1.00
Maximum slope of baseline:	1.00
Minimum peak height:	1.00
Minimum peak area:	100.00
Evaluation interval:	15.00 mm to 135.00 mm
Distance run:	Start: 16.00 mm Front: 135.00 mm
Number of components:	1
Number of standards:	8
Number of samples:	6
Unit of result:	ng
Conversions factor:	1.00
Fractional digits for standards:	1
Fractional digits for samples:	1
Type of calibration function:	$y = a * x$
Calibrate via peak height/area:	Peak height

Lane assignment

No.	Type	Name	Weight [mg]	Solvent [ml]	Dilution	Application vol. [µl]
1	Standard 1	Quercetine	0.1000	0.50	0.00	10.00
2	Standard 2	Rutin	0.1000	0.50	0.00	10.00
3	Standard 3	Stigma sterol	0.1000	0.50	0.00	10.00
4	Standard 4	Gallic acid	0.1000	0.50	0.00	10.00
5	Standard 5	Ellagic acid	0.1000	0.50	0.00	10.00
6	Standard 6	Catechine	0.1000	0.50	0.00	10.00

Date: 28-Nov-13 — 04:04:50 PM   ID: 04798-1385671510-2   Method: Method for Chromatogram

7	Standard 7	Epicatechin	0.1000	0.50	0.00	10.00
8	Standard 8	Piperine	0.1000	0.50	0.00	10.00
9	Sample 1	f1	0.1000	0.50	0.00	10.00
10	Sample 2	f2	0.1000	0.50	0.00	10.00
11	Sample 3	f3	0.1000	0.50	0.00	10.00
12	Sample 4	f4	0.1000	0.50	0.00	10.00
13	Sample 5	f5	0.1000	0.50	0.00	10.00
14	Sample 6	f6	0.1000	0.50	0.00	10.00

Standard concentrations			
Standard	Component name		Concentration
Standard 1	1	: Component 1	0.00 ng
Standard 2	1	: Component 1	0.00 ng
Standard 3	1	: Component 1	0.00 ng
Standard 4	1	: Component 1	0.00 ng
Standard 5	1	: Component 1	0.00 ng
Standard 6	1	: Component 1	0.00 ng
Standard 7	1	: Component 1	0.00 ng
Standard 8	1	: Component 1	0.00 ng

Peak assignment			
Component name	Position [mm]	- Tolerance [mm]	+ Tolerance [mm]
1 : Component 1	0.0	0.0	0.0

Standard and polyherbal solution preparation for fingerprinting at 254 nm

Chapter 5

Results and Observations

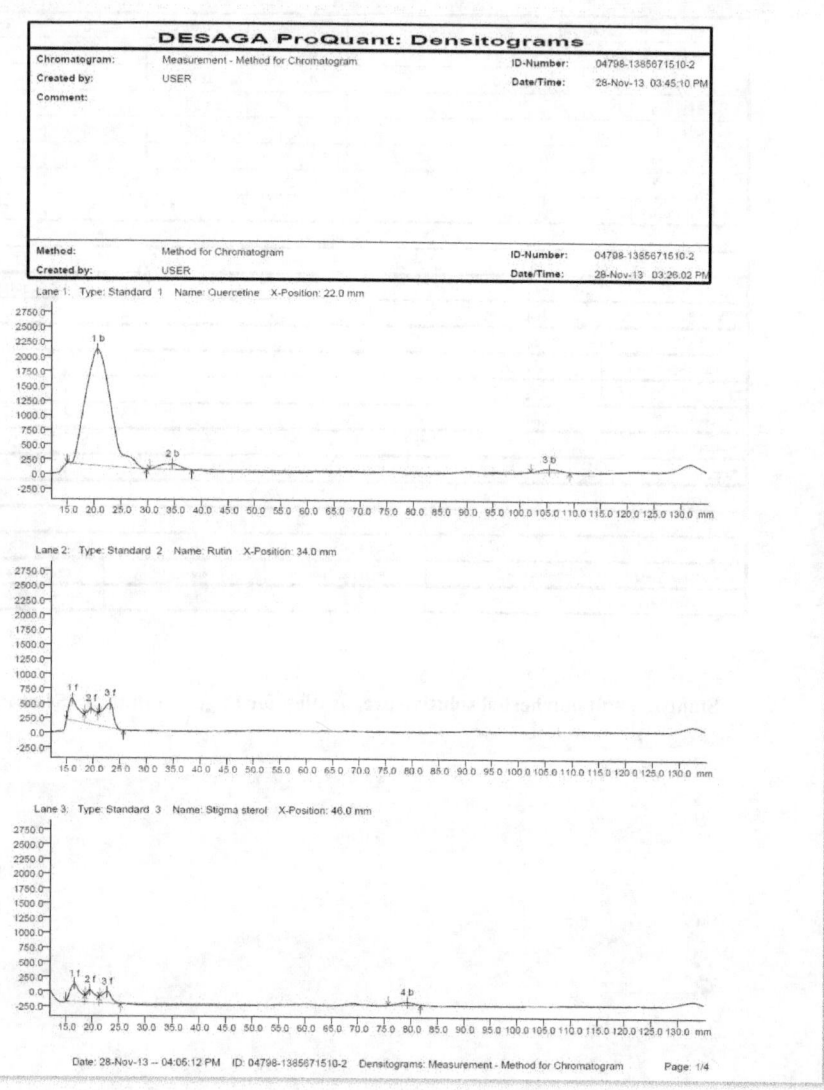

Figure: 5.4: Chromatogram of Standard Quercetin, Rutin and Stigma sterol at 254 nm

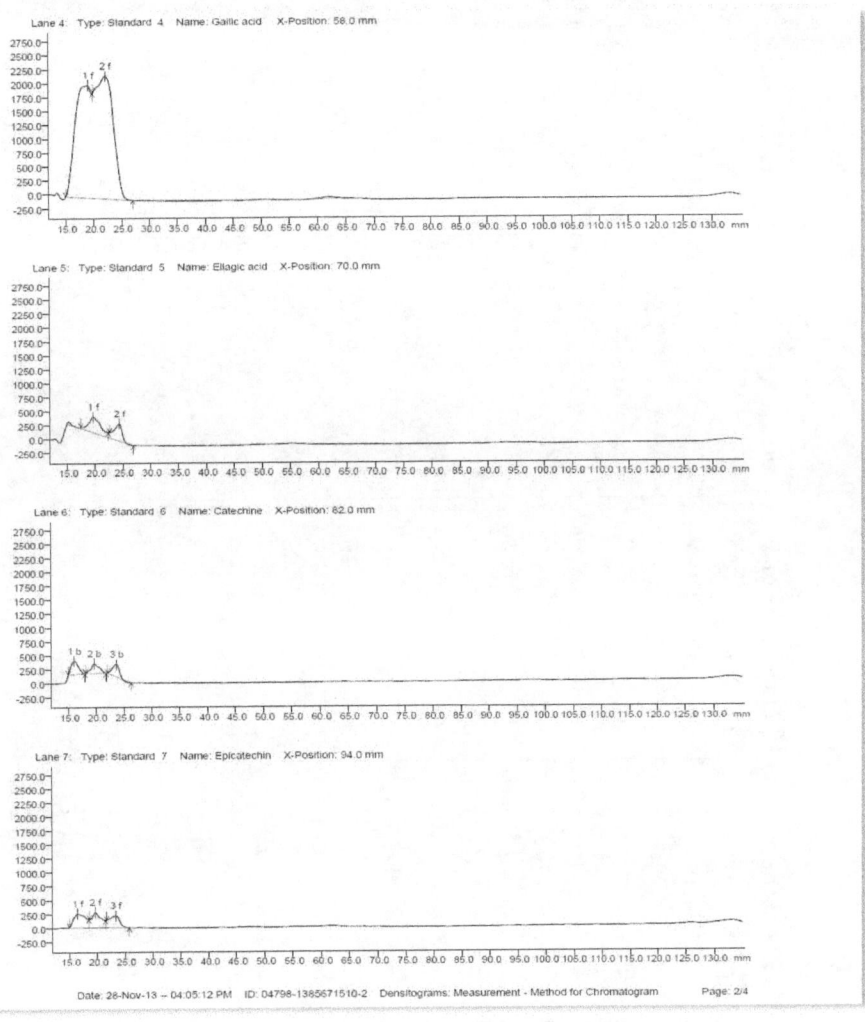

Figure 5.5: Chromatogram of Standard Gallic acid, Ellagic acid, Catechin and Epicatechin at 254 nm

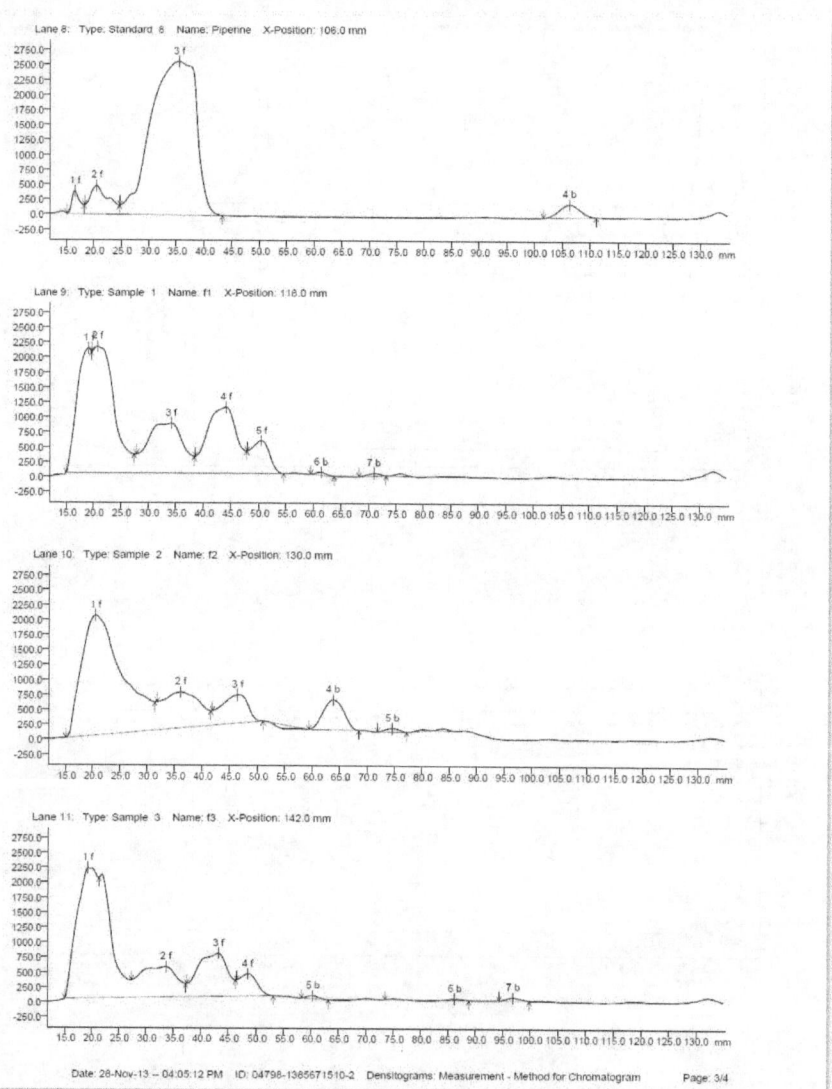

Figure 5.6: Chromatogram of Standard Piperine, Polyherbal FA (f1), FB (f2) and FC (f3) at 254 nm

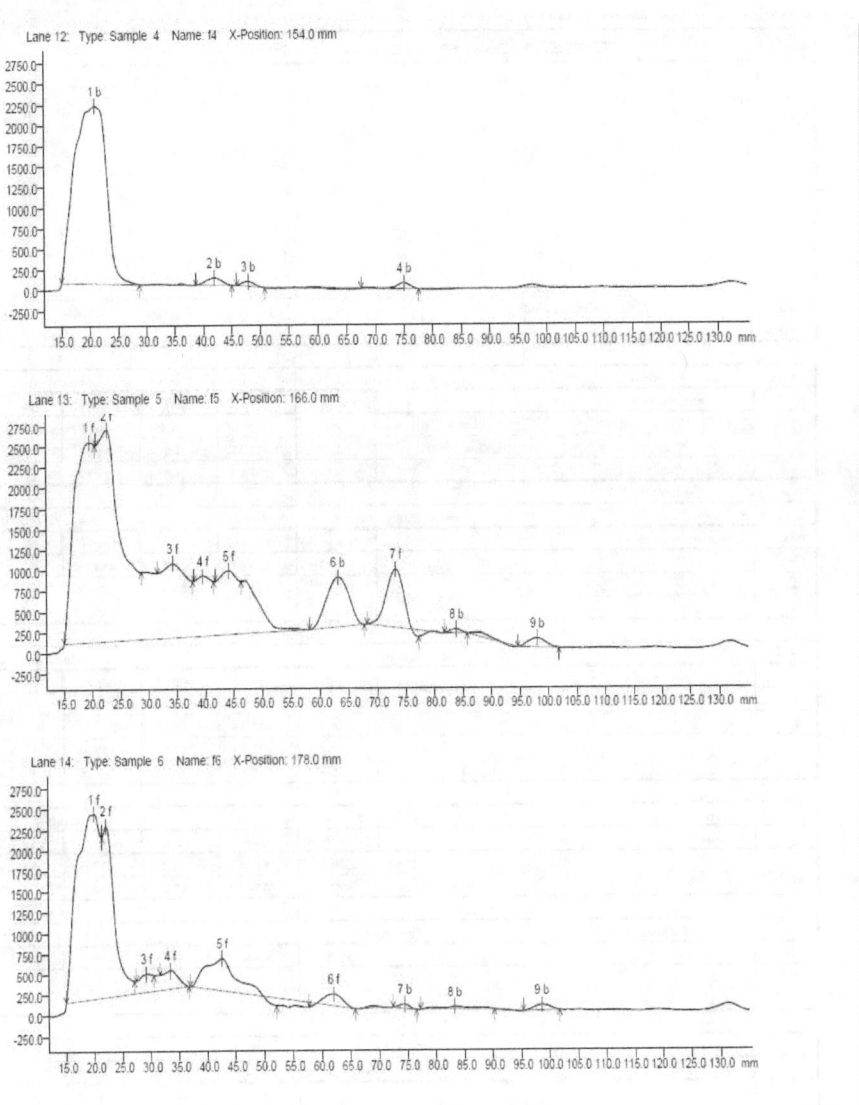

Figure 5.7: Chromatogram of Polyherbal FD (f4), FE (f5) and FF (f6) at 254 nm

DESAGA ProQuant: Peak list

Chromatogram:	Measurement - Method for Chromatogram		ID-Number:	04798-1385671510-2
Created by:	USER		Date/Time:	28-Nov-13 03:45:10 PM
Comment:				

Method:	Method for Chromatogram		ID-Number:	04798-1385671510-2
Created by:	USER		Date/Time:	28-Nov-13 03:26:02 PM

Lane: 1   Type: Standard 1   Name: Quercetin   X-Position: 22.0 mm

Peak	Component name		y-Pos [mm]	Area	Area[%]	Height	Type	Rf
1	:		20.7	10655.50	94.4	1969.67	b	0.04
2	:	Quercetin	34.6	428.06	3.8	95.68	b	0.16
3	:		105.4	207.93	1.8	51.19	b	0.75

Lane: 2   Type: Standard 2   Name: Rutin   X-Position: 34.0 mm

Peak	Component name		y-Pos [mm]	Area	Area[%]	Height	Type	Rf
1	:		16.1	805.85	35.2	381.11	f	0.00
2	:		19.7	528.73	23.1	276.46	f	0.03
3	:	Rutin	23.2	954.06	41.7	416.56	f	0.06

Lane: 3   Type: Standard 3   Name: Stigma sterol   X-Position: 46.0 mm

Peak	Component name		y-Pos [mm]	Area	Area[%]	Height	Type	Rf
1	:		16.7	656.57	42.4	308.30	f	0.01
2	:		19.7	363.36	23.5	217.25	f	0.03
3	:		22.9	378.84	24.5	194.08	f	0.06
4	:	Stigma sterol	79.3	148.64	9.6	46.65	b	0.53

Lane: 4   Type: Standard 4   Name: Gallic acid   X-Position: 58.0 mm

Peak	Component name		y-Pos [mm]	Area	Area[%]	Height	Type	Rf
1	:		19.0	6629.54	44.2	2015.32	f	0.03
2	:	Gallic acid	22.1	8354.15	55.8	2194.08	f	0.05

Lane: 5   Type: Standard 5   Name: Ellagic acid   X-Position: 70.0 mm

Peak	Component name		y-Pos [mm]	Area	Area[%]	Height	Type	Rf
1	:		19.7	700.55	58.8	278.13	f	0.03
2	:	Ellagic acid	24.4	491.09	41.2	302.50	f	0.07

Lane: 6   Type: Standard 6   Name: Catechine   X-Position: 82.0 mm

Peak	Component name		y-Pos [mm]	Area	Area[%]	Height	Type	Rf
1	:		16.1	362.97	37.8	236.62	b	0.00
2	:		19.7	284.39	29.6	169.93	b	0.03
3	:	Catechine	23.7	312.80	32.6	219.44	b	0.06

Chapter 5 — Results and Observations

Lane: 7	Type: Standard 7		Name: Epicatechin				X-Position: 94.0 mm		
Peak	Component name			y-Pos [mm]	Area	Area[%]	Height	Type	Rf
1	:			16.5	602.72	37.8	242.13	f	0.00
2	:			19.7	532.85	33.4	272.93	f	0.03

Date: 28-Nov-13 -- 04:05:30 PM   ID: 04798-1385671510-2   Peak list: Measurement - Method for Chromatogram   Page: 1/3

3	:		Epicatechin	23.4	458.61	28.8	209.74	f	0.06

Lane: 8	Type: Standard 8		Name: Piperine				X-Position: 106.0 mm		
Peak	Component name			y-Pos [mm]	Area	Area[%]	Height	Type	Rf
1	:			16.6	650.43	2.3	381.06	f	0.01
2	:			20.6	1832.94	6.6	474.38	f	0.04
3	:		Piperine	35.5	24433.42	87.8	2559.09	f	0.16
4	:			106.3	922.59	3.3	214.86	b	0.76

Figure 5.8: Peak list of standard compound at 254 nm

Lane: 9 Type: Sample 1 Name: f1 X-Position: 118.0 mm

Peak	Component name	y-Pos [mm]	Area	Area[%]	Height	Type	Rf
1	:	19.2	6026.74	19.4	2080.88	f	0.03
2	: Gallic acid	20.8	9494.21	30.6	2112.67	f	0.04
3	: Quercetin , piperine	34.2	6296.00	20.3	832.10	f	0.15
4	:	44.1	6851.06	22.1	1105.44	f	0.24
5	:	50.5	2125.01	6.9	544.02	f	0.29
6	:	61.4	103.89	0.3	49.66	b	0.38
7	:	71.0	119.43	0.4	45.27	b	0.46

Lane: 10 Type: Sample 2 Name: f2 X-Position: 130.0 mm

Peak	Component name	y-Pos [mm]	Area	Area[%]	Height	Type	Rf
1	: Gallic acid	20.6	17442.37	64.1	1995.83	f	0.04
2	: Quercetin , piperine	36.1	4753.42	17.5	599.73	f	0.16
3	:	46.4	2650.80	9.7	473.83	f	0.26
4	:	63.6	2184.90	8.0	501.97	b	0.40
5	:	74.6	171.74	0.6	56.22	b	0.49

Lane: 11 Type: Sample 3 Name: f3 X-Position: 142.0 mm

Peak	Component name	y-Pos [mm]	Area	Area[%]	Height	Type	Rf
1	:	19.3	9513.90	48.0	2166.65	f	0.03
2	: Quercetin , piperine	33.6	3986.27	20.1	504.20	f	0.15
3	:	43.2	4568.34	23.1	719.46	f	0.23
4	:	48.5	1385.41	7.0	372.35	f	0.27
5	:	60.4	117.72	0.6	49.01	b	0.37
6	: Stigma sterol	86.2	104.17	0.5	25.51	b	0.59
7	:	96.9	140.31	0.7	48.76	b	0.68

Lane: 12 Type: Sample 4 Name: f4 X-Position: 154.0 mm

Peak	Component name	y-Pos [mm]	Area	Area[%]	Height	Type	Rf
1	: Gallic acid	20.9	14005.19	95.8	2145.74	b	0.04
2	:	41.8	281.93	1.9	89.26	b	0.22
3	:	47.9	144.88	1.0	58.37	b	0.27
4	: Stigma sterol	75.0	188.64	1.3	67.59	b	0.50

Lane: 13 Type: Sample 5 Name: f5 X-Position: 166.0 mm

Peak	Component name	y-Pos [mm]	Area	Area[%]	Height	Type	Rf
1	: Gallic acid	19.5	9542.66	24.9	2411.79	f	0.04
2	: Rutin, Ellagic acid, Catechin, Epicatechin	22.6	12659.75	33.1	2550.88	f	0.06
3	: Quercetin, piperine	34.2	4918.81	12.8	895.01	f	0.15
4	:	39.5	2355.59	6.2	721.33	f	0.20
5	:	44.1	3183.65	8.3	770.08	f	0.24
6	:	63.1	2690.41	7.0	598.18	b	0.40
7	:	73.2	2442.16	6.4	704.37	f	0.48

Chapter 5 — Results and Observations

8	:	Stigma sterol	83.8	100.62	0.3	46.42	b	0.57
9	:		98.0	404.03	1.1	112.50	b	0.69

Lane: 14	Type: Sample 6		Name: f6				X-Position: 178.0 mm	
Peak	Component name			y-Pos [mm]	Area	Area[%]	Height	Type	Rf
1	:			20.0	10639.69	51.7	2235.91	f	0.03
2	:	Gallic acid		22.1	5025.27	24.4	2069.45	f	0.05
3	:			29.2	599.04	2.9	222.96	f	0.11
4	:	Quercetin, piperine		33.4	722.28	3.5	225.41	f	0.15
5	:			42.6	2510.85	12.2	389.33	f	0.22
6	:			62.0	509.80	2.5	140.21	f	0.39
7	:			74.4	100.35	0.5	48.82	b	0.49
8	:	Stigma sterol		83.2	235.90	1.1	32.52	b	0.56
9	:			98.5	222.27	1.1	65.79	b	0.69

Figure 5.9: Peak list of Polyherbal Formulations at 254 nm

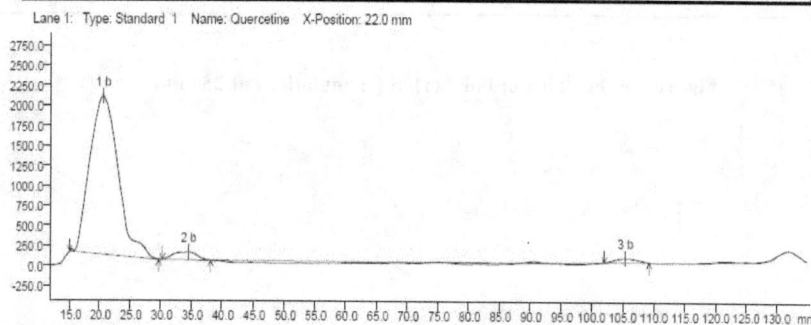

Figure 5.10: Chromatogram of Quercetin at 254 nm

Chapter 5 — Results and Observations

DESAGA ProQuant: Densitogram + Peaklist

Chromatogram:	Measurement - Method for Chromatogram	ID-Number:	04798-1385671510-2
Created by:	USER	Date/Time:	28-Nov-13 03:45:10 PM
Comment:			

Method:	Method for Chromatogram	ID-Number:	04798-1385671510-2
Created by:	USER	Date/Time:	28-Nov-13 03:26:02 PM

Lane 2: Type: Standard 2 Name: Rutin X-Position: 34.0 mm

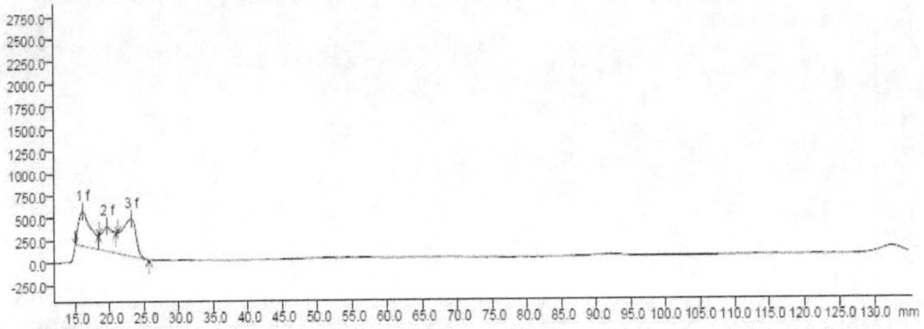

Lane: 2	Type: Standard 2	Name: Rutin				X-Position: 34.0 mm		
Peak	Component name		y-Pos [mm]	Area	Area[%]	Height	Type	Rf
1	:		16.1	805.85	35.2	381.11	f	0.00
2	:		19.7	528.73	23.1	276.46	f	0.03
3	:		23.2	954.06	41.7	416.56	f	0.06

Figure 5.11: Chromatogram of Rutin at 254 nm

DESAGA ProQuant: Densitogram + Peaklist

Chromatogram:	Measurement - Method for Chromatogram	ID-Number:	04798-1385671510-2
Created by:	USER	Date/Time:	28-Nov-13 03:45:10 PM
Comment:			

Method:	Method for Chromatogram	ID-Number:	04798-1385671510-2
Created by:	USER	Date/Time:	28-Nov-13 03:26:02 PM

Lane: 3 Type: Standard 3 Name: Stigma sterol X-Position: 46.0 mm

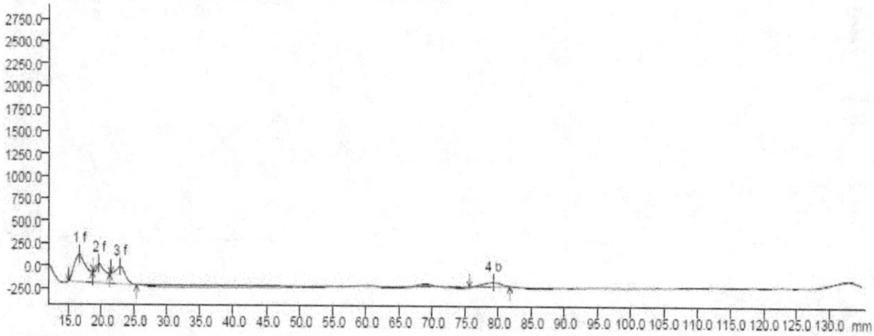

Lane: 3 Type: Standard 3 Name: Stigma sterol X-Position: 46.0 mm

Peak	Component name	y-Pos [mm]	Area	Area[%]	Height	Type	Rf
1	:	16.7	656.57	42.4	308.30	f	0.01
2	:	19.7	363.36	23.5	217.25	f	0.03
3	:	22.9	378.84	24.5	194.08	f	0.06
4	:	79.3	148.64	9.6	46.65	b	0.53

Figure 5.12: Chromatogram of Stigma sterol at 254 nm

Chapter 5 — Results and Observations

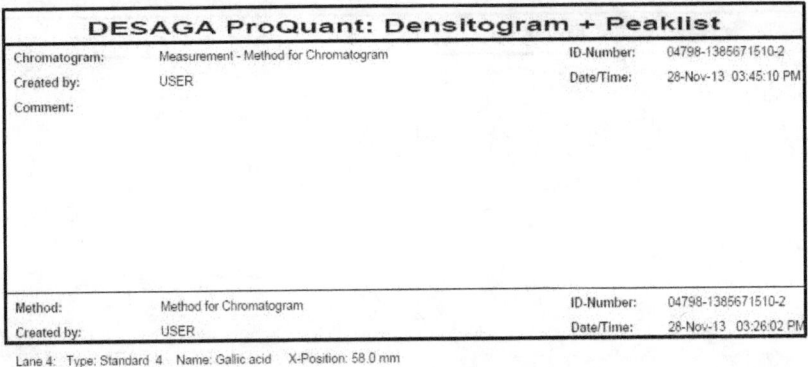

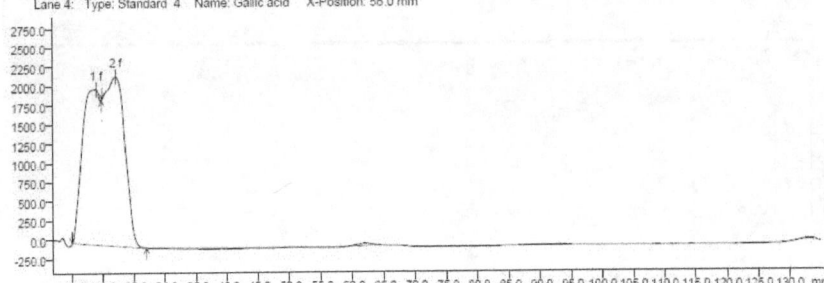

Lane: 4	Type: Standard 4		Name: Gallic acid				X-Position: 58.0 mm		
Peak	Component name			y-Pos [mm]	Area	Area[%]	Height	Type	Rf
1	:			19.0	6629.54	44.2	2015.32	f	0.03
2	:			22.1	8354.15	55.8	2194.08	f	0.05

Figure 5.13: Chromatogram of Gallic acid at 254 nm

DESAGA ProQuant: Densitogram + Peaklist

Chromatogram:	Measurement - Method for Chromatogram	ID-Number:	04798-1385671510-2
Created by:	USER	Date/Time:	28-Nov-13 03:45:10 PM
Comment:			

Method:	Method for Chromatogram	ID-Number:	04798-1385671510-2
Created by:	USER	Date/Time:	28-Nov-13 03:26:02 PM

Lane 5: Type: Standard 5   Name: Ellagic acid   X-Position: 70.0 mm

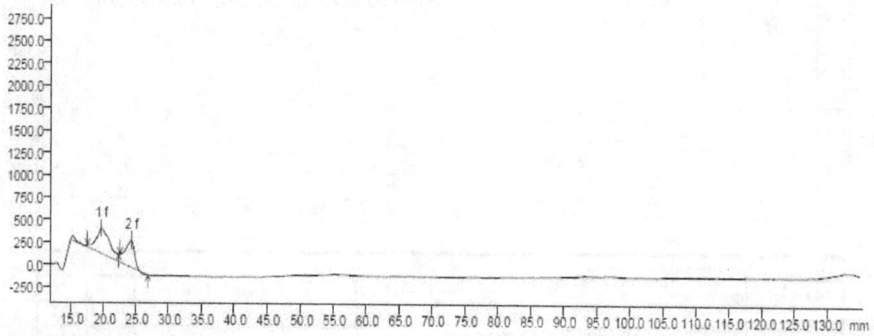

Lane: 5	Type: Standard 5	Name: Ellagic acid			X-Position: 70.0 mm		
Peak	Component name	y-Pos [mm]	Area	Area[%]	Height	Type	Rf
1	;	19.7	700.55	58.8	278.13	f	0.03
2	;	24.4	491.09	41.2	302.50	f	0.07

Figure 5.14: Chromatogram of Ellagic acid at 254 nm

Chapter 5   Results and Observations

DESAGA ProQuant: Densitogram + Peaklist

Chromatogram:	Measurement - Method for Chromatogram	ID-Number:	04798-1385671510-2
Created by:	USER	Date/Time:	28-Nov-13 03:45:10 PM
Comment:			

Method:	Method for Chromatogram	ID-Number:	04798-1385671510-2
Created by:	USER	Date/Time:	28-Nov-13 03:26:02 PM

Lane: 6 Type: Standard 6 Name: Catechine X-Position: 82.0 mm

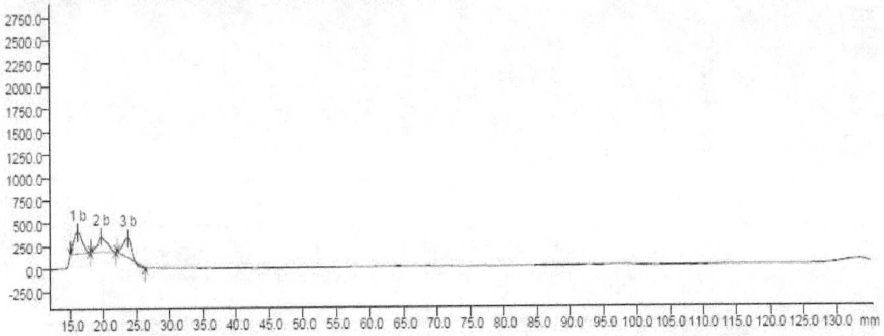

Lane: 6 Type: Standard 6 Name: Catechine X-Position: 82.0 mm

Peak	Component name	y-Pos [mm]	Area	Area[%]	Height	Type	Rf
1	:	16.1	362.97	37.8	236.62	b	0.00
2	:	19.7	284.39	29.6	169.93	b	0.03
3	:	23.7	312.80	32.6	219.44	b	0.06

Figure 5.15: Chromatogram of Catechin at 254 nm

Chapter 5

Results and Observations

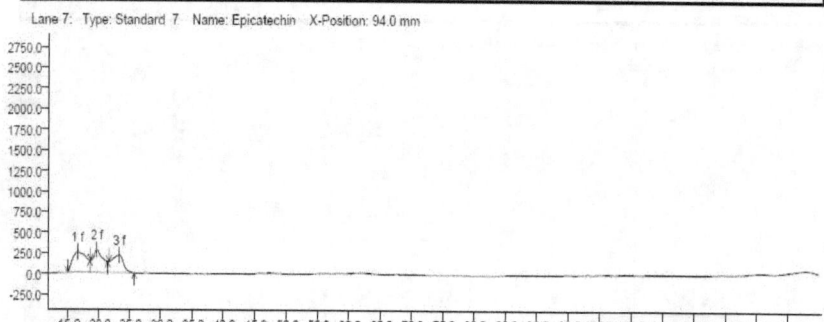

Figure 5.16: Chromatogram of Epicatechin at 254 nm

Chapter 5 — Results and Observations

DESAGA ProQuant: Densitogram + Peaklist

Chromatogram:	Measurement - Method for Chromatogram	ID-Number:	04798-1385671510-2
Created by:	USER	Date/Time:	28-Nov-13 03:45:10 PM
Comment:			

Method:	Method for Chromatogram	ID-Number:	04798-1385671510-2
Created by:	USER	Date/Time:	28-Nov-13 03:26:02 PM

Lane 8: Type: Standard 8 Name: Piperine X-Position: 106.0 mm

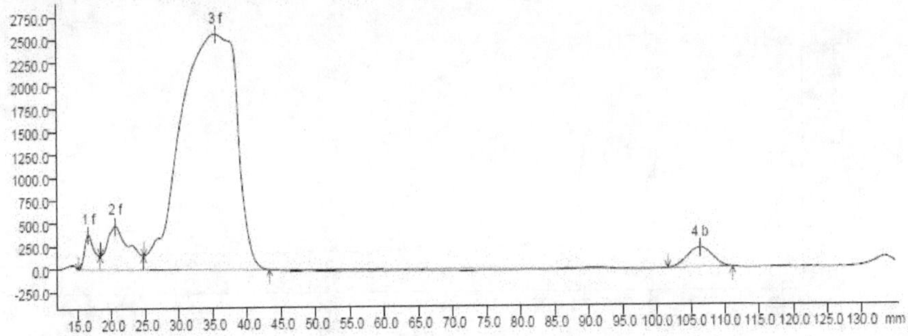

Lane: 8   Type: Standard 8   Name: Piperine   X-Position: 106.0 mm

Peak	Component name	y-Pos [mm]	Area	Area[%]	Height	Type	Rf
1	:	16.6	650.43	2.3	381.06	f	0.01
2	:	20.6	1832.94	6.6	474.38	f	0.04
3	:	35.5	24433.42	87.8	2559.09	f	0.16
4	:	106.3	922.59	3.3	214.86	b	0.76

Figure 5.17: Chromatogram of Piperine at 254 nm

DESAGA ProQuant: Densitogram + Peaklist

Chromatogram:	Measurement - Method for Chromatogram	**ID-Number:**	04798-1385671510-2
Created by:	USER	**Date/Time:**	28-Nov-13 03:45:10 PM
Comment:			
Method:	Method for Chromatogram	**ID-Number:**	04798-1385671510-2
Created by:	USER	**Date/Time:**	28-Nov-13 03:26:02 PM

Lane 9: Type: Sample 1 Name: f1 X-Position: 118.0 mm

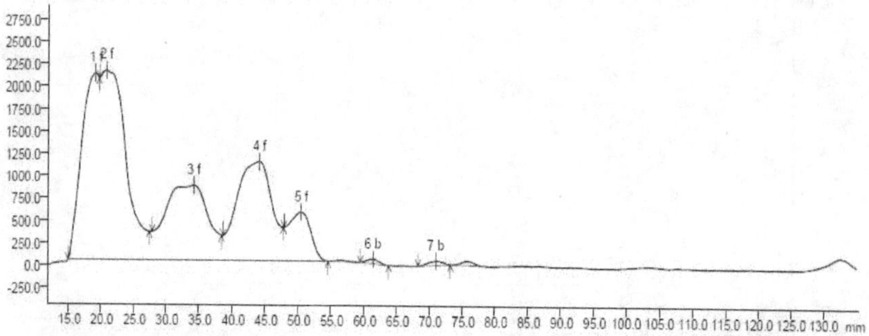

Lane: 9	Type: Sample 1	Name: f1				X-Position: 118.0 mm	
Peak	**Component name**	**y-Pos [mm]**	**Area**	**Area[%]**	**Height**	**Type**	**Rf**
1	:	19.2	6026.74	19.4	2080.88	f	0.03
2	:	20.8	9494.21	30.6	2112.67	f	0.04
3	:	34.2	6296.00	20.3	832.10	f	0.15
4	:	44.1	6851.06	22.1	1105.44	f	0.24
5	:	50.5	2125.01	6.9	544.02	f	0.29
6	:	61.4	103.89	0.3	49.66	b	0.38
7	:	71.0	119.43	0.4	45.27	b	0.46

Figure 5.18: Chromatogram of Polyherbal formulation FA (f1) at 254 nm

Chapter 5 — Results and Observations

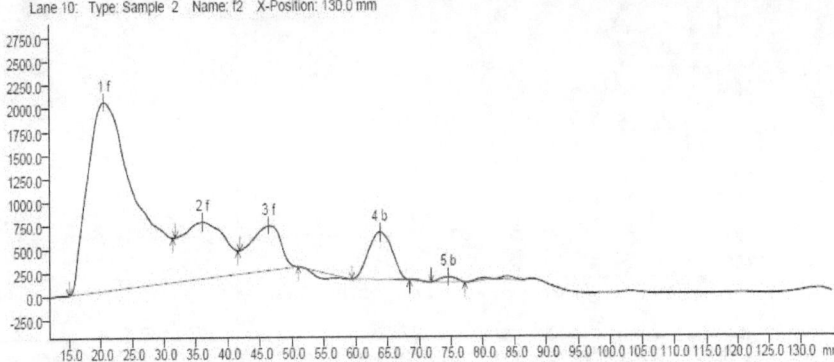

Figure 5.19: Chromatogram of Polyherbal formulation FB (f2) at 254 nm

Chapter 5 Results and Observations

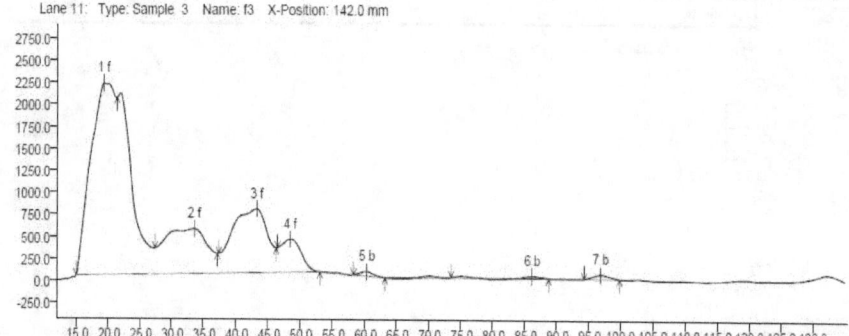

Figure 5.20: Chromatogram of Polyherbal formulation FC (f3) at 254 nm

Chapter 5 — Results and Observations

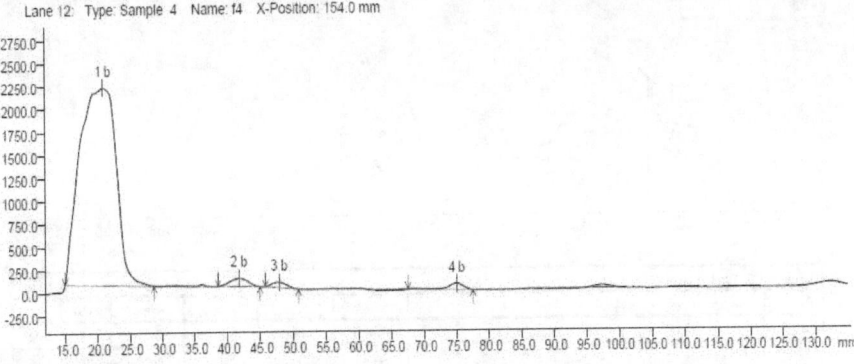

Figure 5.21: Chromatogram of Polyherbal formulation FD (f4) at 254 nm

Chapter 5 — Results and Observations

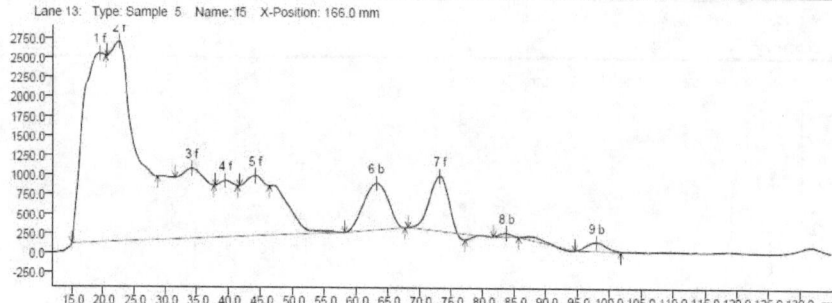

Figure 5.22: Chromatogram of Polyherbal formulation FE (f5) at 254 nm

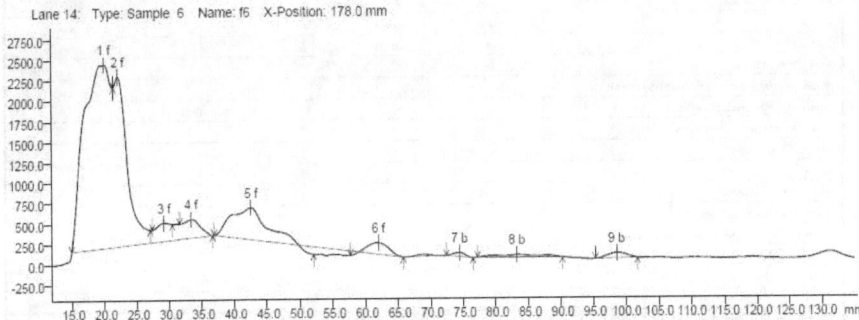

Figure 5.23: Chromatogram of Polyherbal formulation FF (f6) at 254 nm

DESAGA ProQuant: Method for chromatogram

Name of Method:	Method for Chromatogram
Created by:	USER
Comment:	
Date/Time:	28-Nov-13 03:26:02 PM

Start coordinate X:	22.0 mm	Slit width:	4.00 mm
Start coordinate Y:	11.0 mm	Slit height:	0.40 mm
End coordinate Y:	135.0 mm	Wavelength:	366 nm
Number of lanes:	14	Wavelength (Reference):	0 nm
Distance of lanes:	12.0 [mm]	Filter position:	Open
Mode:	Remission	Signal:	positive
Evaluation mode:	Extinction	Lamp:	Deu/Tungsten

Maeander width:	0.0 mm
Subsoil correction for maeanderscan:	no
Resolution at measurement:	0.100 mm
Number of measurements/point:	1
Smoothing value:	None
Lane optimization:	no
Automatic zeroing:	yes
Signal range of graphic:	-1000 to 1000
Autom. evaluation after measurement:	yes
Window width:	1.00 mm
Threshold for peak detection:	0.00
Maximum slope of baseline:	1.00
Minimum peak height:	4.00
Minimum peak area:	5.00
Evaluation interval:	20.00 mm to 135.00 mm
Distance run:	Start: 16.00 mm Front: 135.00 mm
Number of components:	1
Number of standards:	8
Number of samples:	8
Unit of result:	ng
Conversions factor:	1.00
Fractional digits for standards:	1
Fractional digits for samples:	1
Type of calibration function:	y = a * x
Calibrate via peak height/area:	Peak height

Lane assignment

No.	Type	Name	Weight [mg]	Solvent [ml]	Dilution	Application vol. [µl]
1	Standard 1	Quercetine	0.1000	0.50	0.00	10.00
2	Standard 2	Rutin	0.1000	0.50	0.00	10.00
3	Standard 3	Stigma sterol	0.1000	0.50	0.00	10.00
4	Standard 4	Gallic acid	0.1000	0.50	0.00	10.00
5	Standard 5	Ellagic acid	0.1000	0.50	0.00	10.00
6	Standard 6	Catechine	0.1000	0.50	0.00	10.00

Chapter 5
Results and Observations

			0.1000	0.50	0.00	10.00
7	Standard 7	Epicatechin	0.1000	0.50	0.00	10.00
8	Standard 8	Piperine	0.1000	0.50	0.00	10.00
9	Sample 1	f1	0.1000	0.50	0.00	10.00
10	Sample 2	f2	0.1000	0.50	0.00	10.00
11	Sample 3	f3	0.1000	0.50	0.00	10.00
12	Sample 4	f4	0.1000	0.50	0.00	10.00
13	Sample 5	f5	0.1000	0.50	0.00	10.00
14	Sample 6	f6	0.1000	0.50	0.00	10.00

Standard concentrations		
Standard	Component name	Concentration
Standard 1	1 : Component 1	0.00 ng
Standard 2	1 : Component 1	0.00 ng
Standard 3	1 : Component 1	0.00 ng
Standard 4	1 : Component 1	0.00 ng
Standard 5	1 : Component 1	0.00 ng
Standard 6	1 : Component 1	0.00 ng
Standard 7	1 : Component 1	0.00 ng
Standard 8	1 : Component 1	0.00 ng

Peak assignment			
Component name	Position [mm]	- Tolerance [mm]	+ Tolerance [mm]
1 : Component 1	0.0	0.0	0.0

Standard and polyherbal solution preparation for fingerprinting at 366 nm

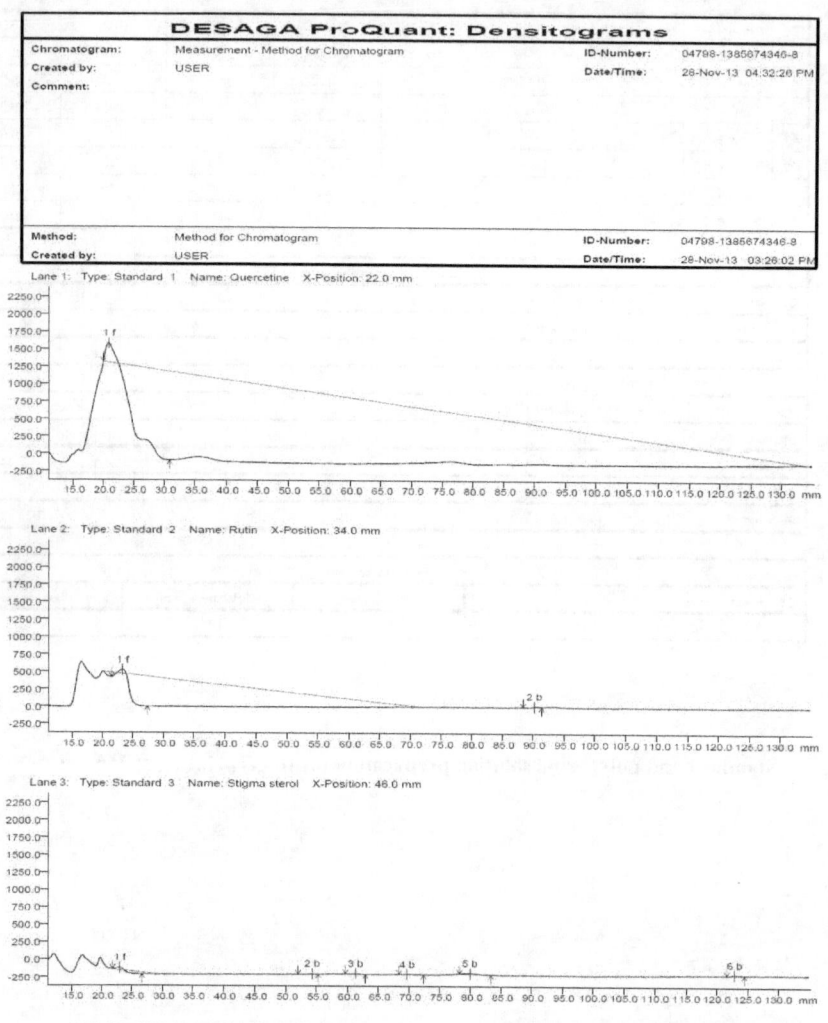

Figure 5.24: Chromatogram of Standard Quercetin, Rutin and Stigma sterol at 366 nm

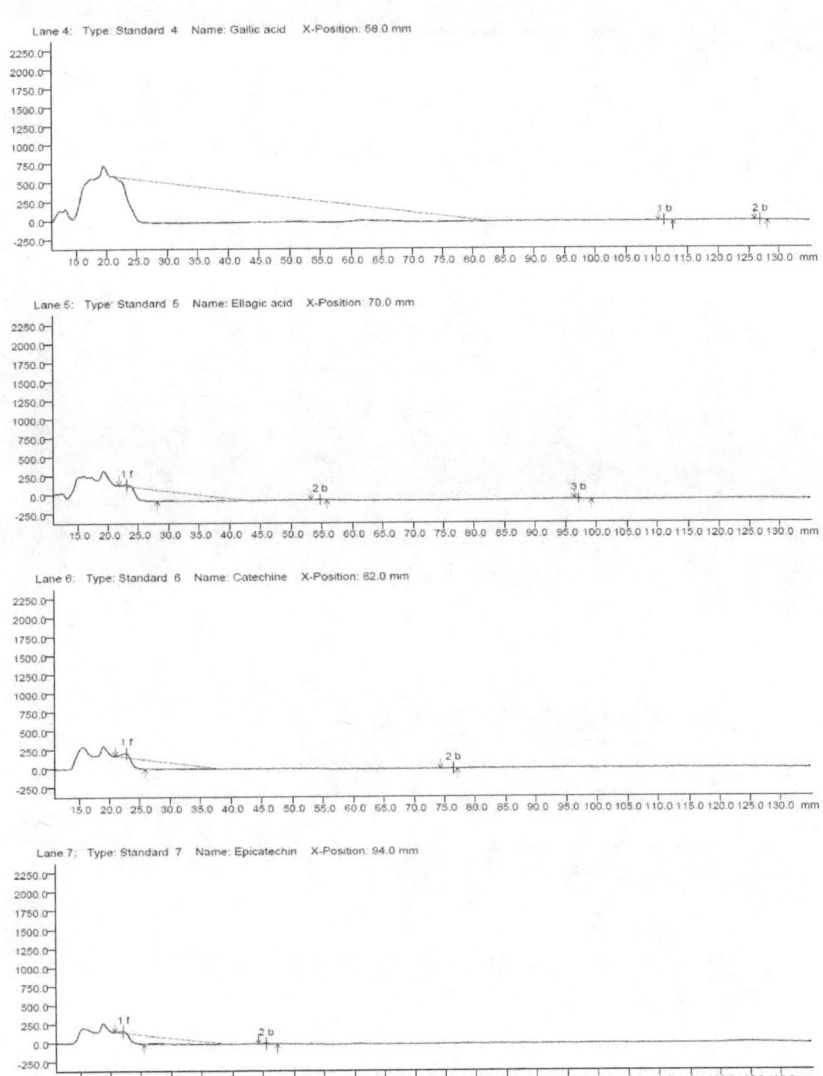

Figure 5.25: Chromatogram of Gallic acid, Ellagic acid, Catechin and Epicatechin at 366 nm

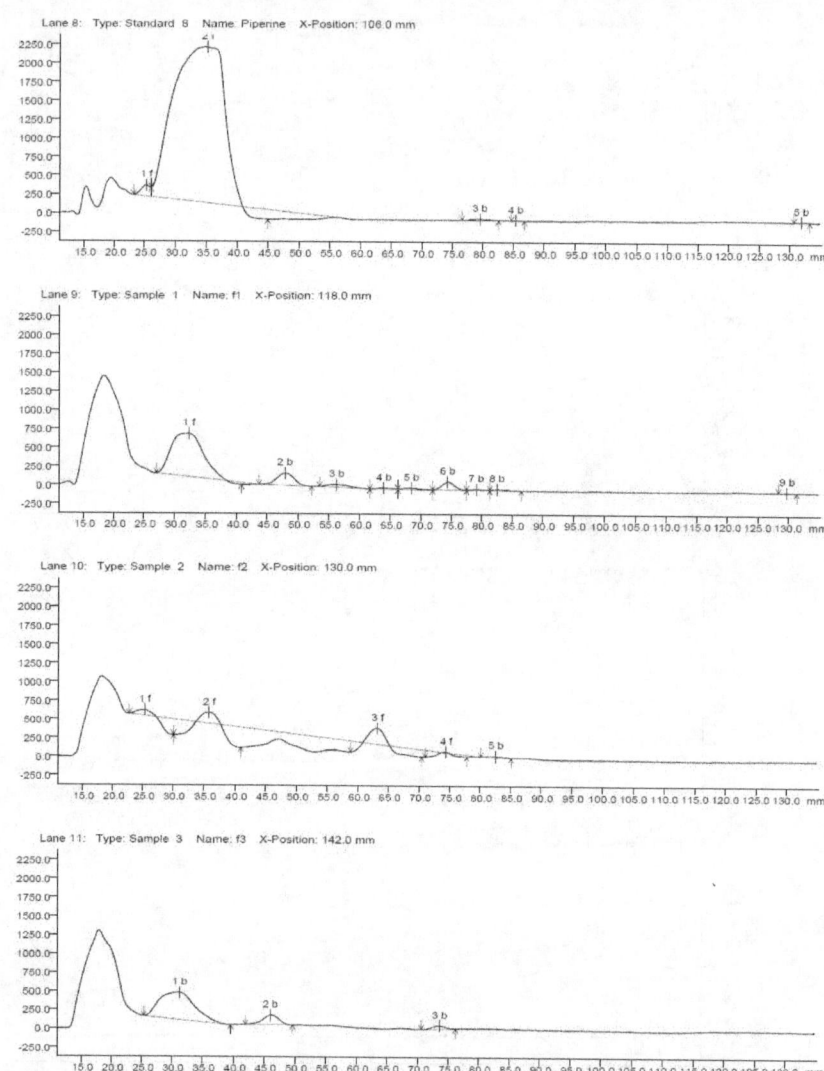

Figure 5.26: Chromatogram of Piperine, Polyherbal FA (f1), FB (f2) and FC (f3) at 366 nm

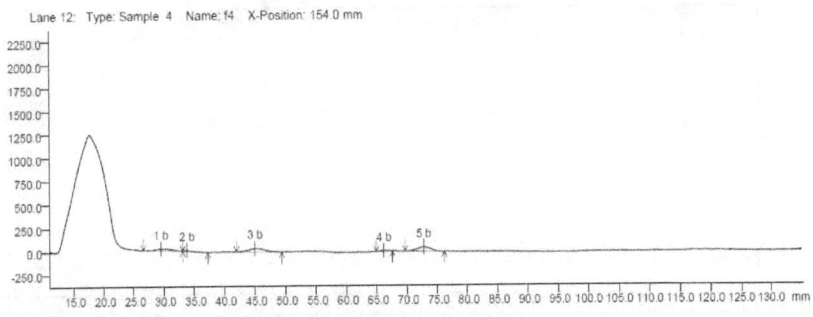
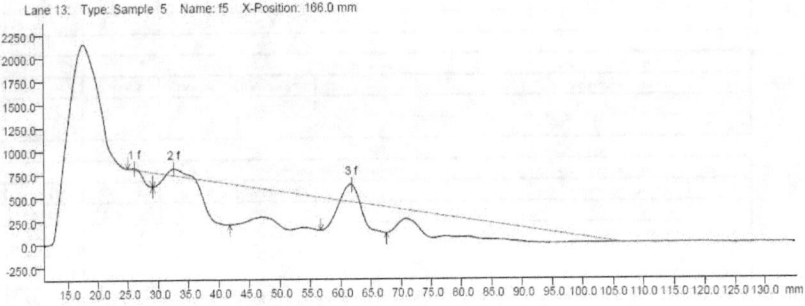
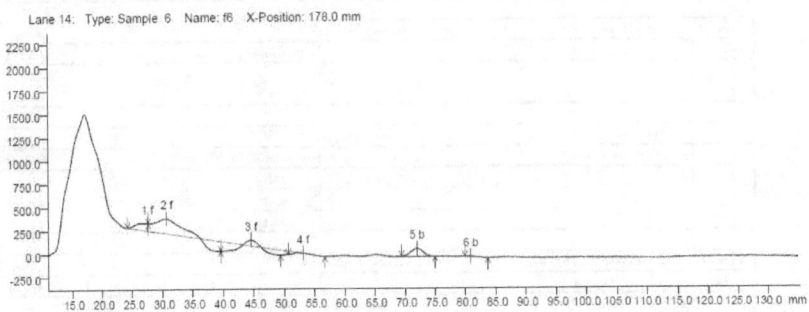

Figure 5.27: Chromatogram of Polyherbal FD (f4), FE (f5) and FF (f6) at 366 nm

DESAGA ProQuant: Peak list

Chromatogram:	Measurement - Method for Chromatogram	ID-Number:	04798-1385674346-8
Created by:	USER	Date/Time:	28-Nov-13 04:32:26 PM
Comment:			

Method:	Method for Chromatogram	ID-Number:	04798-1385674346-8
Created by:	USER	Date/Time:	28-Nov-13 03:26:02 PM

Lane: 1   Type: Standard 1   Name: Quercetine   X-Position: 22.0 mm

Peak	Component name		y-Pos [mm]	Area	Area[%]	Height	Type	Rf
1	:	Quercetine	20.9	392.67	100.0	273.62	f	0.04

Lane: 2   Type: Standard 2   Name: Rutin   X-Position: 34.0 mm

Peak	Component name		y-Pos [mm]	Area	Area[%]	Height	Type	Rf
1	:	Rutin	23.3	51.15	87.8	52.43	f	0.06
2	:		90.2	7.10	12.2	5.30	b	0.62

Lane: 3   Type: Standard 3   Name: Stigma sterol   X-Position: 46.0 mm

Peak	Component name		y-Pos [mm]	Area	Area[%]	Height	Type	Rf
1	:		23.0	34.16	36.2	32.15	f	0.06
2	:		54.3	7.36	7.8	5.06	b	0.32
3	:		61.3	13.88	14.7	8.57	b	0.38
4	:		69.7	6.08	6.5	4.27	b	0.45
5	:	Stigma sterol	79.9	24.38	25.9	11.28	b	0.54
6	:		122.9	8.42	8.9	8.17	b	0.90

Lane: 4   Type: Standard 4   Name: Gallic acid   X-Position: 58.0 mm

Peak	Component name		y-Pos [mm]	Area	Area[%]	Height	Type	Rf
1	:	Gallic acid	111.3	5.56	51.5	4.86	b	0.80
2	:		126.9	5.24	48.5	4.83	b	0.93

Lane: 5   Type: Standard 5   Name: Ellagic acid   X-Position: 70.0 mm

Peak	Component name		y-Pos [mm]	Area	Area[%]	Height	Type	Rf
1	:	Ellagic acid	23.1	32.04	71.3	21.98	f	0.06
2	:		54.7	6.36	14.2	5.82	b	0.33
3	:		97.1	6.55	14.6	7.20	b	0.68

Lane: 6   Type: Standard 6   Name: Catechine   X-Position: 82.0 mm

Peak	Component name		y-Pos [mm]	Area	Area[%]	Height	Type	Rf
1	:	Catechine	22.8	77.53	92.5	57.39	f	0.06
2	:		76.4	6.28	7.5	4.65	b	0.51

Lane: 7   Type: Standard 7   Name: Epicatechin   X-Position: 94.0 mm

Peak	Component name		y-Pos [mm]	Area	Area[%]	Height	Type	Rf
1	:	Epicatechin	22.1	32.01	81.0	27.48	f	0.05
2	:		45.5	7.51	19.0	5.30	b	0.25

Chapter 5 — Results and Observations

Lane: 8 Type: Standard 8 Name: Piperine X-Position: 106.0 mm

Peak	Component name		y-Pos [mm]	Area	Area[%]	Height	Type	Rf
1	:		25.3	239.72	1.2	144.99	f	0.08
2	:	Piperine	35.1	19774.60	98.5	2073.45	f	0.16
3	:		79.5	43.13	0.2	14.82	b	0.53
4	:		85.4	6.33	0.0	7.58	b	0.58
5	:		131.9	6.83	0.0	6.45	b	0.97

Lane: 9 Type: Sample 1 Name: f1 X-Position: 118.0 mm

Peak	Component name		y-Pos [mm]	Area	Area[%]	Height	Type	Rf
1	:	Piperine	32.3	3403.19	76.5	575.82	f	0.14
2	:		47.9	525.47	11.8	164.19	b	0.27
3	:		56.3	141.84	3.2	33.75	b	0.34
4	:		64.0	31.59	0.7	12.98	b	0.40
5	:		68.5	47.56	1.1	18.49	b	0.44
6	:		74.4	252.10	5.7	105.64	b	0.49
7	:		79.1	13.90	0.3	8.19	b	0.53
8	:	Stigma sterol	82.5	26.83	0.6	11.02	b	0.56
9	:		129.8	7.92	0.2	5.70	b	0.96

Lane: 10 Type: Sample 2 Name: f2 X-Position: 130.0 mm

Peak	Component name		y-Pos [mm]	Area	Area[%]	Height	Type	Rf
1	:	Rutin, Ellagic acid, Catechin	25.3	205.33	17.1	75.53	f	0.08
2	:	Piperine	35.8	377.96	31.4	145.30	f	0.17
3	:		63.2	573.74	47.7	214.30	f	0.40
4	:		74.4	9.64	0.8	11.65	f	0.49
5	:	Stigma sterol	82.6	37.36	3.1	13.26	b	0.56

Lane: 11 Type: Sample 3 Name: f3 X-Position: 142.0 mm

Peak	Component name		y-Pos [mm]	Area	Area[%]	Height	Type	Rf
1	:	Piperine	31.3	2399.80	83.1	360.96	b	0.13
2	:		46.0	386.99	13.4	125.85	b	0.25
3	:		73.6	101.94	3.5	43.23	b	0.48

Lane: 12 Type: Sample 4 Name: f4 X-Position: 154.0 mm

Peak	Component name		y-Pos [mm]	Area	Area[%]	Height	Type	Rf
1	:		29.5	64.21	20.3	20.51	b	0.11
2	:	Piperine	33.8	7.15	2.3	9.71	b	0.15
3	:		45.0	109.98	34.7	37.40	b	0.24
4	:		66.2	12.26	3.9	7.18	b	0.42
5	:		72.8	123.22	38.9	45.75	b	0.48

Lane: 13 Type: Sample 5 Name: f5 X-Position: 166.0 mm

Peak	Component name		y-Pos [mm]	Area	Area[%]	Height	Type	Rf
1	:	Rutin, Ellagic acid, Catechin	26.1	17.14	2.8	16.09	f	0.08
2	:	Piperine	32.6	210.85	34.3	73.99	f	0.14
3	:		61.8	386.63	62.9	184.44	f	0.38

Lane: 14 Type: Sample 6 Name: f6 X-Position: 178.0 mm

Peak	Component name		y-Pos [mm]	Area	Area[%]	Height	Type	Rf
1	:		27.5	169.94	12.5	78.61	f	0.10
2	:	Piperine	30.7	847.95	62.5	160.76	f	0.12
3	:		44.6	117.25	8.6	63.12	f	0.24
4	:		53.1	9.42	0.7	5.20	f	0.31
5	:		72.0	201.72	14.9	86.84	b	0.47
6	:	Stigma sterol	80.9	10.82	0.8	6.61	b	0.55

Figure 5.28: Peak list of Standards and Polyherbal Formulations at 366 nm

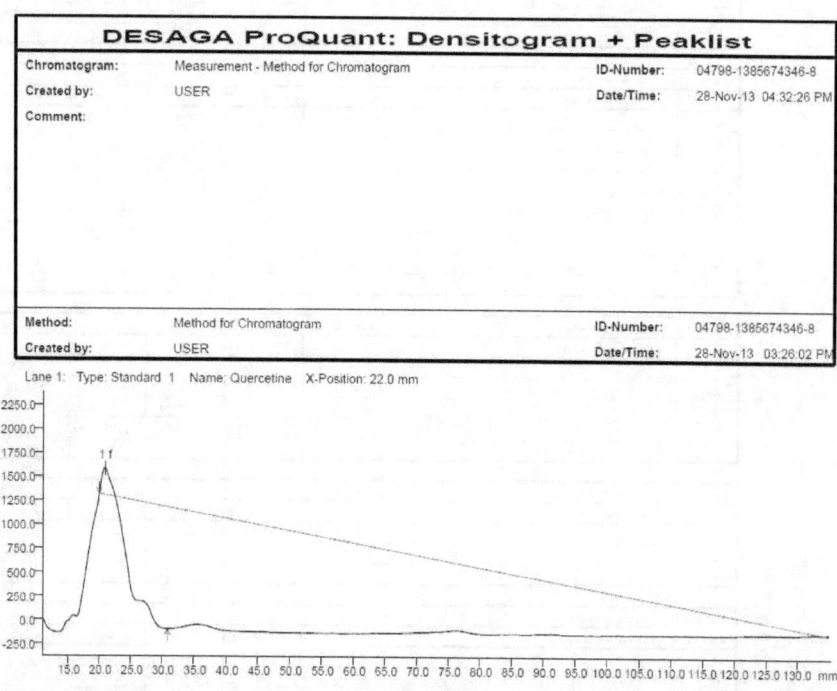

Figure 5.29: Chromatogram of Quercetin at 366 nm

Chapter 5 — Results and Observations

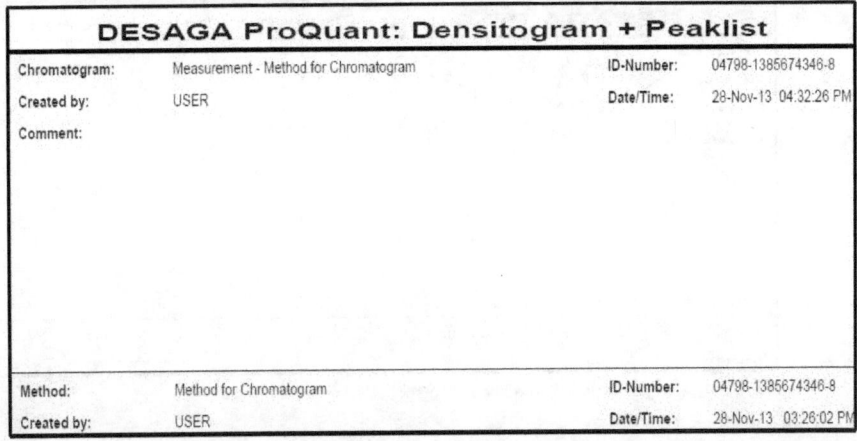

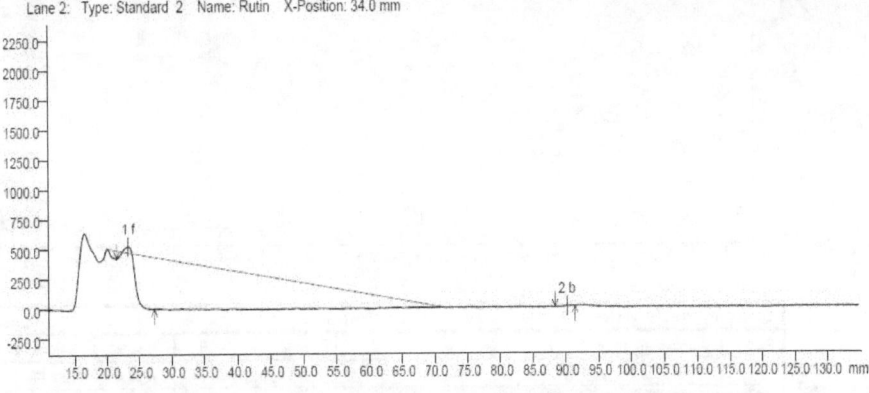

Lane: 2	Type: Standard 2		Name: Rutin				X-Position: 34.0 mm	
Peak	Component name		y-Pos [mm]	Area	Area[%]	Height	Type	Rf
1	:		23.3	51.15	87.8	52.43	f	0.06
2	:		90.2	7.10	12.2	5.30	b	0.62

Figure 5.30: Chromatogram of Rutin at 366 nm

Chapter 5 — Results and Observations

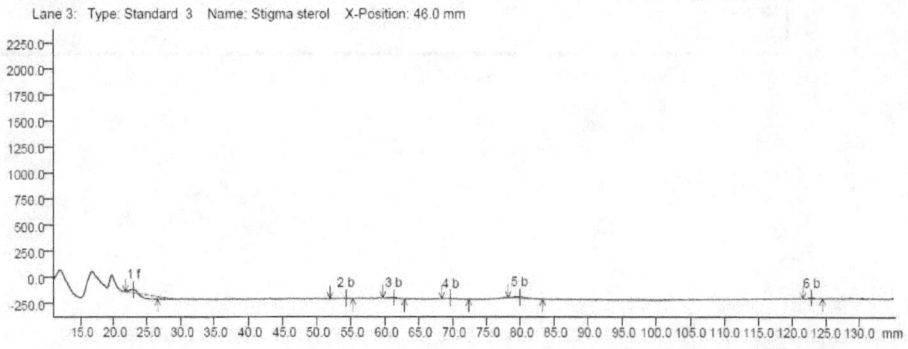

Figure 5.31: Chromatogram of Stigma sterol at 366 nm

Chapter 5   *Results and Observations*

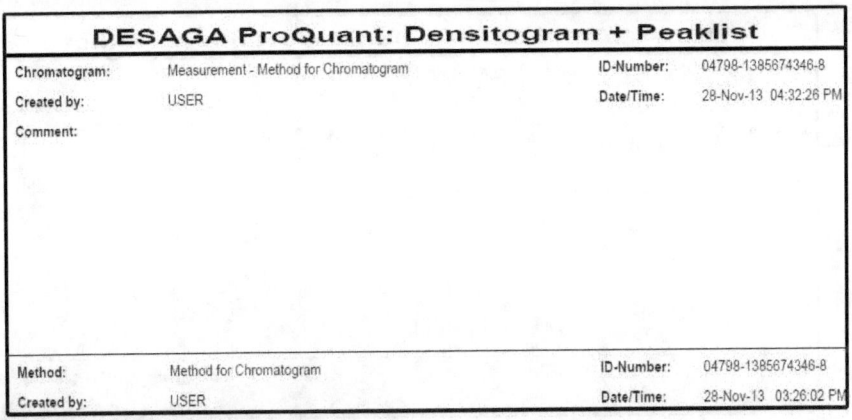

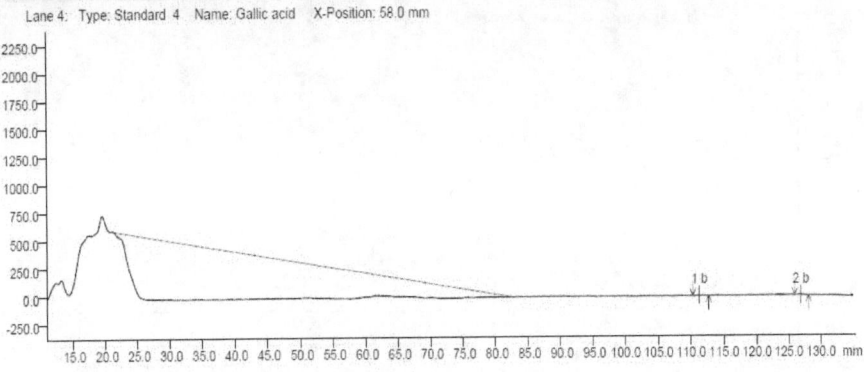

Figure 5.32: Chromatogram of Gallic acid at 366 nm

Chapter 5
Results and Observations

DESAGA ProQuant: Densitogram + Peaklist

Chromatogram:	Measurement - Method for Chromatogram	ID-Number:	04798-1385674346-8
Created by:	USER	Date/Time:	28-Nov-13 04:32:26 PM
Comment:			

Method:	Method for Chromatogram	ID-Number:	04798-1385674346-8
Created by:	USER	Date/Time:	28-Nov-13 03:26:02 PM

Lane 5: Type: Standard 5 Name: Ellagic acid X-Position: 70.0 mm

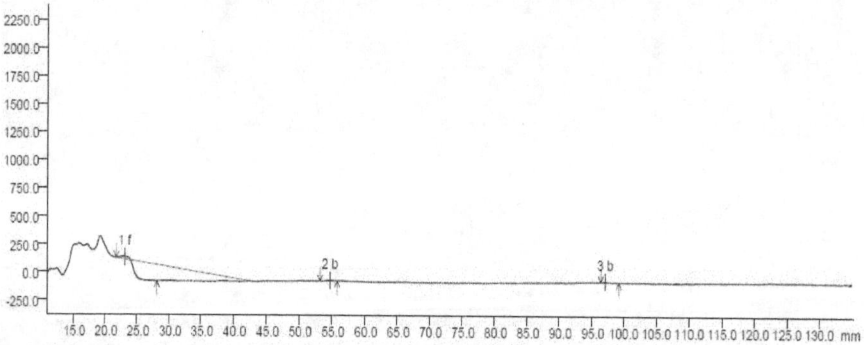

Lane: 5	Type: Standard 5		Name: Ellagic acid				X-Position: 70.0 mm	
Peak	Component name		y-Pos [mm]	Area	Area[%]	Height	Type	Rf
1	:		23.1	32.04	71.3	21.98	f	0.06
2	:		54.7	6.36	14.2	5.82	b	0.33
3	:		97.1	6.55	14.6	7.20	b	0.68

Figure 5.33: Chromatogram of Ellagic acid at 366 nm

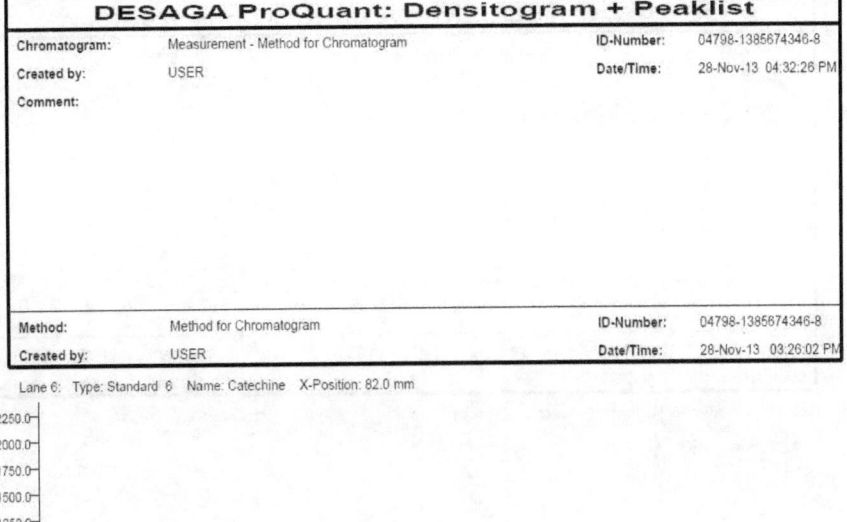

Figure 5.34: Chromatogram of Catechin at 366 nm

DESAGA ProQuant: Densitogram + Peaklist

Chromatogram:	Measurement - Method for Chromatogram	ID-Number:	04798-1385674346-8
Created by:	USER	Date/Time:	28-Nov-13 04:32:26 PM
Comment:			

Method:	Method for Chromatogram	ID-Number:	04798-1385674346-8
Created by:	USER	Date/Time:	28-Nov-13 03:26:02 PM

Lane: 7 Type: Standard 7 Name: Epicatechin X-Position: 94.0 mm

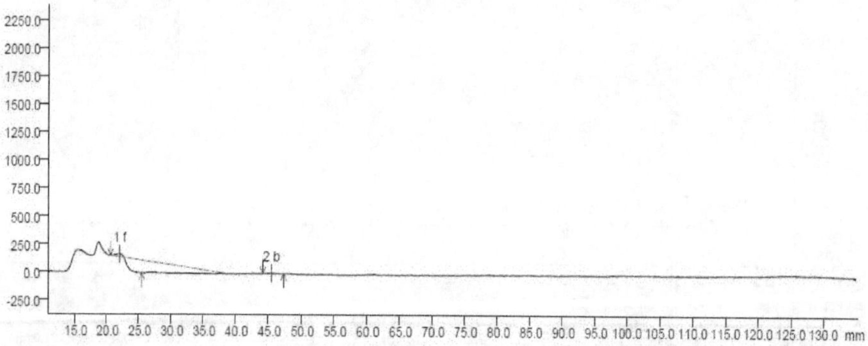

Lane: 7 Type: Standard 7 Name: Epicatechin X-Position: 94.0 mm

Peak	Component name	y-Pos [mm]	Area	Area[%]	Height	Type	Rf
1	:	22.1	32.01	81.0	27.48	f	0.05
2	:	45.5	7.51	19.0	5.30	b	0.25

Figure 5.35: Chromatogram of Epicatechin at 366 nm

Chapter 5

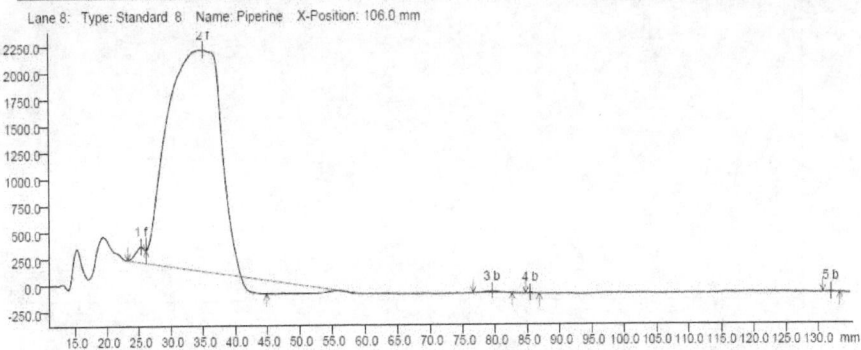

Figure 5.36: Chromatogram of Piperine at 366 nm

Chapter 5 — Results and Observations

DESAGA ProQuant: Densitogram + Peaklist

Chromatogram:	Measurement - Method for Chromatogram	ID-Number:	04798-1385674346-8
Created by:	USER	Date/Time:	28-Nov-13 04:32:26 PM
Comment:			

Method:	Method for Chromatogram	ID-Number:	04798-1385674346-8
Created by:	USER	Date/Time:	28-Nov-13 03:26:02 PM

Lane: 9 Type: Sample 1 Name: f1 X-Position: 118.0 mm

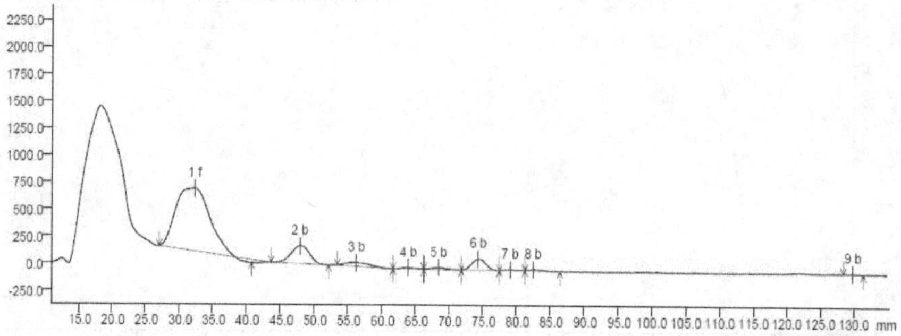

Lane: 9 Type: Sample 1 Name: f1 X-Position: 118.0 mm

Peak	Component name	y-Pos [mm]	Area	Area[%]	Height	Type	Rf
1	:	32.3	3403.19	76.5	575.82	f	0.14
2	:	47.9	525.47	11.8	164.19	b	0.27
3	:	56.3	141.84	3.2	33.75	b	0.34
4	:	64.0	31.59	0.7	12.98	b	0.40
5	:	68.5	47.56	1.1	18.49	b	0.44
6	:	74.4	252.10	5.7	105.64	b	0.49
7	:	79.1	13.90	0.3	8.19	b	0.53
8	:	82.5	26.83	0.6	11.02	b	0.56
9	:	129.8	7.92	0.2	5.70	b	0.96

Figure 5.37: Chromatogram of Polyherbal Formulation FA (f1) at 366 nm

Chapter 5 — Results and Observations

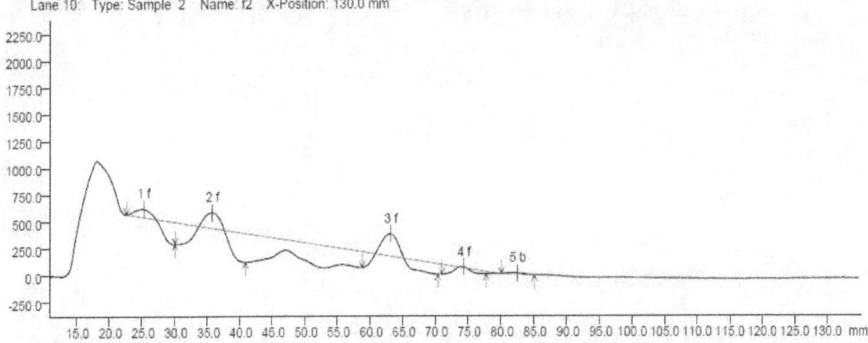

Figure 5.38: Chromatogram of Polyherbal Formulation FB (f2) at 366 nm

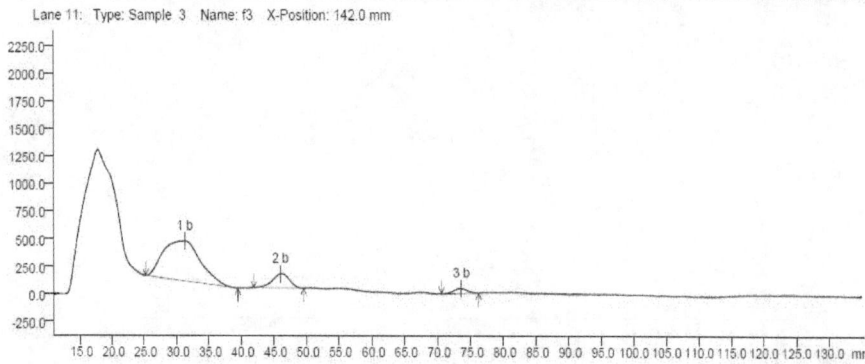

Figure 5.39: Chromatogram of Polyherbal Formulation FC (f3) at 366 nm

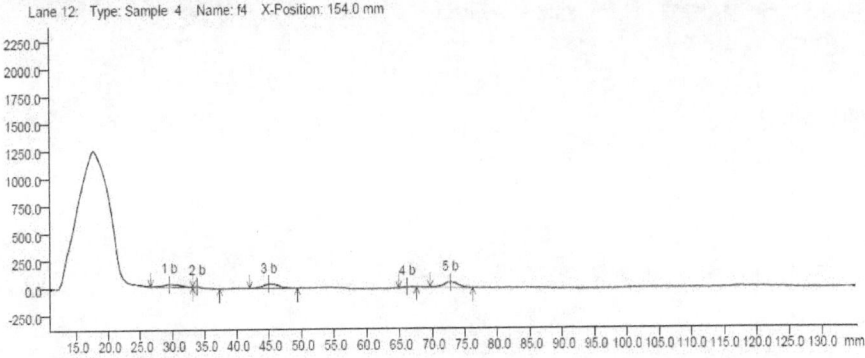

Figure 5.40: Chromatogram of Polyherbal Formulation FD (f4) at 366 nm

DESAGA ProQuant: Densitogram + Peaklist

Chromatogram:	Measurement - Method for Chromatogram	ID-Number:	04798-1385674346-8
Created by:	USER	Date/Time:	28-Nov-13 04:32:26 PM
Comment:			

Method:	Method for Chromatogram	ID-Number:	04798-1385674346-8
Created by:	USER	Date/Time:	28-Nov-13 03:26:02 PM

Lane: 13 Type: Sample 5 Name: f5 X-Position: 166.0 mm

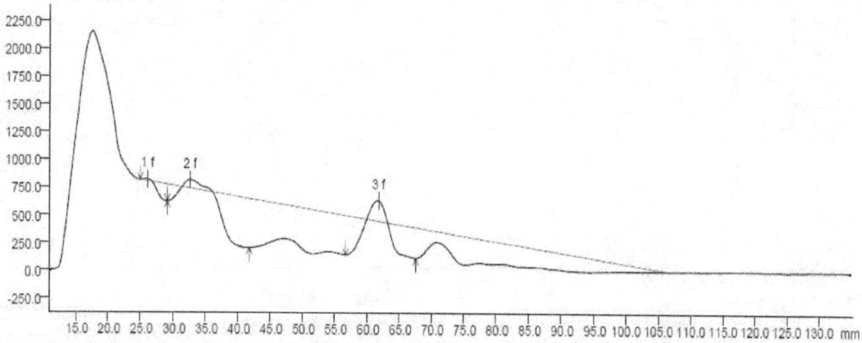

Lane: 13	Type: Sample 5		Name: f5				X-Position: 166.0 mm	
Peak	Component name			y-Pos [mm]	Area	Area[%]	Height	Type	Rf
1	:			26.1	17.14	2.8	16.09	f	0.08
2	:			32.6	210.85	34.3	73.99	f	0.14
3	:			61.8	386.63	62.9	184.44	f	0.38

Figure 5.41: Chromatogram of Polyherbal Formulation FE (f5) at 366 nm

DESAGA ProQuant: Densitogram + Peaklist

Chromatogram:	Measurement - Method for Chromatogram	ID-Number:	04798-1385674346-8
Created by:	USER	Date/Time:	28-Nov-13 04:32:26 PM
Comment:			

Method:	Method for Chromatogram	ID-Number:	04798-1385674346-8
Created by:	USER	Date/Time:	28-Nov-13 03:26:02 PM

Lane 14: Type: Sample 6   Name: f6   X-Position: 178.0 mm

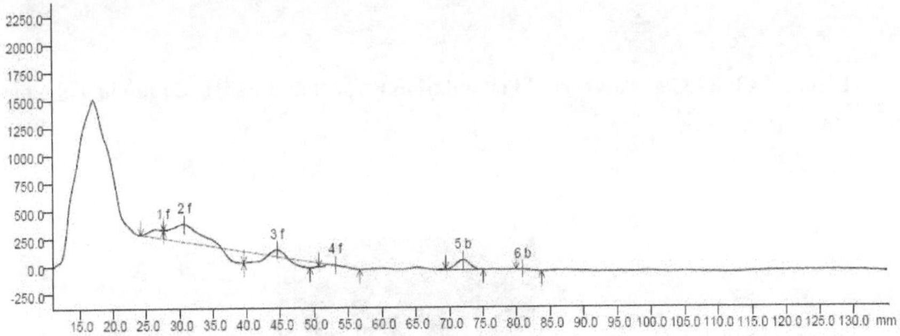

Lane: 14	Type: Sample 6	Name: f6					X-Position: 178.0 mm
Peak	Component name	y-Pos [mm]	Area	Area[%]	Height	Type	Rf
1	:	27.5	169.94	12.5	78.61	f	0.10
2	:	30.7	847.95	62.5	160.76	f	0.12
3	:	44.6	117.25	8.6	63.12	f	0.24
4	:	53.1	9.42	0.7	5.20	f	0.31
5	:	72.0	201.72	14.9	86.84	b	0.47
6	:	80.9	10.82	0.8	6.61	b	0.55

Figure 5.42: Chromatogram of Polyherbal Formulation FF (f6) at 366 nm

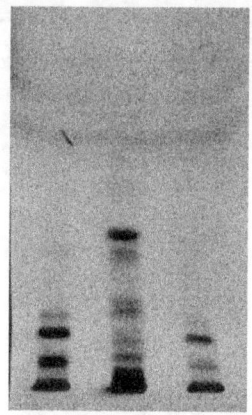

Figure 5.43: TLC of Polyherbal Formulation FA, FB and FC at 254 nm in Toluene: EAA (17:3.5 % v/v)

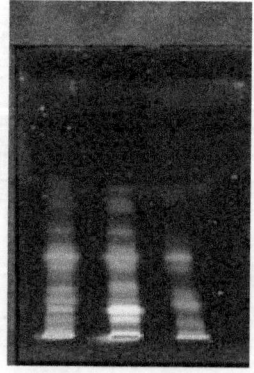

Figure: 5.44: TLC of Polyherbal Formulation FA, FB and FC at 366 nmin Toluene:

EAA (17:3.5 % v/v)

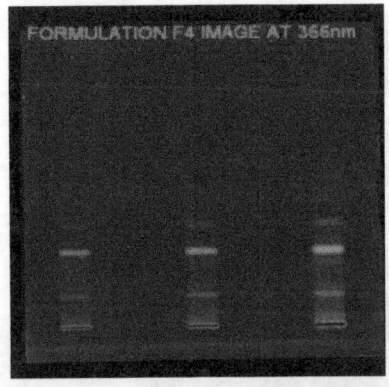 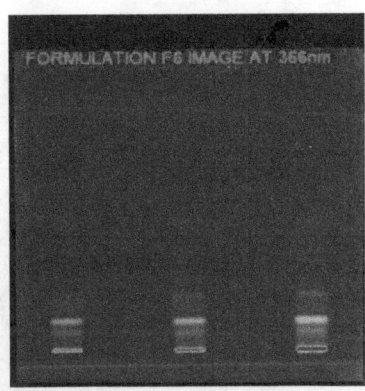

Figure 5.45: TLC of FD(f4) at 366 nm   **Figure 5.46: TLC of FE (f5) at 366 nm**

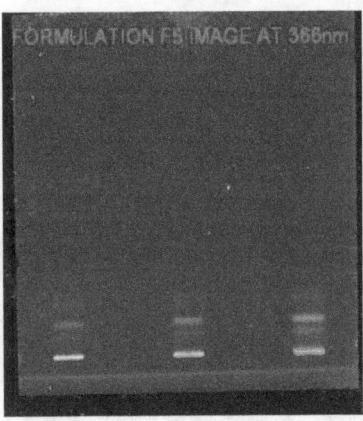

Figure 5.47: TLC of FF(f6) at 366 nm

Mobile Phase: Toluene: EAA (17:3.5 % v/v)

Figure 5.48: TLC of Polyherbal Formulations with standards at 254 nm in Toluene: EAA (17:3.5 % v/v)

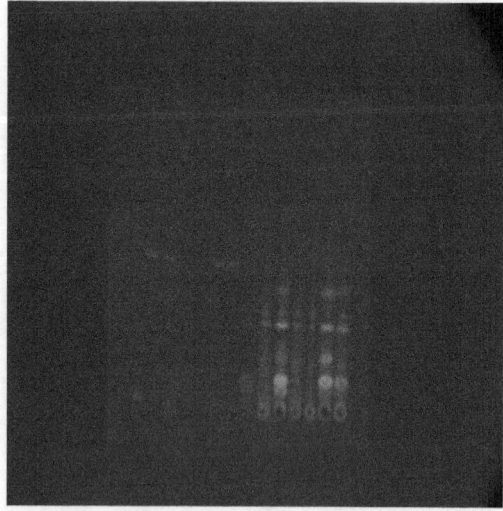

Figure 5.49: TLC of Polyherbal Formulations with standards at 366 nm in Toluene:

EAA (17:3.5 % v/v)

DESAGA ProQuant: Method for chromatogram

Name of Method:	Method for Chromatogram
Created by:	USER
Comment:	
Date/Time:	29-Nov-13 12:20:57 PM

Start coordinate X:	22.0 mm	Slit width:	4.00 mm
Start coordinate Y:	10.0 mm	Slit height:	0.40 mm
End coordinate Y:	135.0 mm	Wavelength:	420 nm
Number of lanes:	14	Wavelength (Reference):	0 nm
Distance of lanes:	10.0 [mm]	Filter position:	Open
Mode:	Remission	Signal:	positive
Evaluation mode:	Extinction	Lamp:	Deu/Tungsten

Maeander width:	0.0 mm
Subsoil correction for maeanderscan:	no
Resolution at measurement:	0.100 mm
Number of measurements/point:	1
Smoothing value:	None
Lane optimization:	no
Automatic zeroing:	yes
Signal range of graphic:	-1000 to 1000
Autom. evaluation after measurement:	yes
Window width:	1.00 mm
Threshold for peak detection:	0.00
Maximum slope of baseline:	1.00
Minimum peak height:	10.00
Minimum peak area:	10.00
Evaluation interval:	15.00 mm to 135.00 mm
Distance run:	Start: 15.00 mm Front: 135.00 mm
Number of components:	4
Number of standards:	8
Number of samples:	6
Unit of result:	ng
Conversions factor:	1.00
Fractional digits for standards:	1
Fractional digits for samples:	1
Type of calibration function:	$y = a * x$
Calibrate via peak height/area:	Peak height

Lane assignment

No.	Type	Name	Weight [mg]	Solvent [ml]	Dilution	Application vol. [µl]
1	Standard 1	Quercetine	0.1000	0.50	0.00	10.00
2	Standard 2	Rutin	0.1000	0.50	0.00	10.00
3	Standard 3	Stigma sterol	0.1000	0.50	0.00	10.00
4	Standard 4	Gallic acid	0.1000	0.50	0.00	10.00
5	Standard 5	Ellagic acid	0.1000	0.50	0.00	10.00
6	Standard 6	Catechine	0.1000	0.50	0.00	10.00

Chapter 5 — Results and Observations

7	Standard 7	Epicatechine		0.1000	0.50	0.00	10.00
8	Standard 8	Piperine		0.1000	0.50	0.00	10.00
9	Sample 1	f1		0.1000	0.50	0.00	10.00
10	Sample 2	f2		0.1000	0.50	0.00	10.00
11	Sample 3	f3		0.1000	0.50	0.00	10.00
12	Sample 4	f4		0.1000	0.50	0.00	10.00
13	Sample 5	f5		0.1000	0.50	0.00	10.00
14	Sample 6	f6		0.1000	0.50	0.00	10.00

Standard concentrations			
Standard	Component name		Concentration
Standard 1	1	: Component 1	0.00 ng
	2	: Component 2	0.00 ng
	3	: Component 3	0.00 ng
	4	: Component 4	0.00 ng
Standard 2	1	: Component 1	0.00 ng
	2	: Component 2	0.00 ng
	3	: Component 3	0.00 ng
	4	: Component 4	0.00 ng
Standard 3	1	: Component 1	0.00 ng
	2	: Component 2	0.00 ng
	3	: Component 3	0.00 ng
	4	: Component 4	0.00 ng
Standard 4	1	: Component 1	0.00 ng
	2	: Component 2	0.00 ng
	3	: Component 3	0.00 ng
	4	: Component 4	0.00 ng
Standard 5	1	: Component 1	0.00 ng
	2	: Component 2	0.00 ng
	3	: Component 3	0.00 ng
	4	: Component 4	0.00 ng
Standard 6	1	: Component 1	0.00 ng
	2	: Component 2	0.00 ng
	3	: Component 3	0.00 ng
	4	: Component 4	0.00 ng
Standard 7	1	: Component 1	0.00 ng
	2	: Component 2	0.00 ng
	3	: Component 3	0.00 ng
	4	: Component 4	0.00 ng
Standard 8	1	: Component 1	0.00 ng
	2	: Component 2	0.00 ng
	3	: Component 3	0.00 ng
	4	: Component 4	0.00 ng

Peak assignment			
Component name	Position [mm]	- Tolerance [mm]	+ Tolerance [mm]
1 : Component 1	0.0	0.0	0.0
2 : Component 2	0.0	0.0	0.0
3 : Component 3	0.0	0.0	0.0
4 : Component 4	0.0	0.0	0.0

Standard and polyherbal solution preparation for fingerprinting at 420 nm

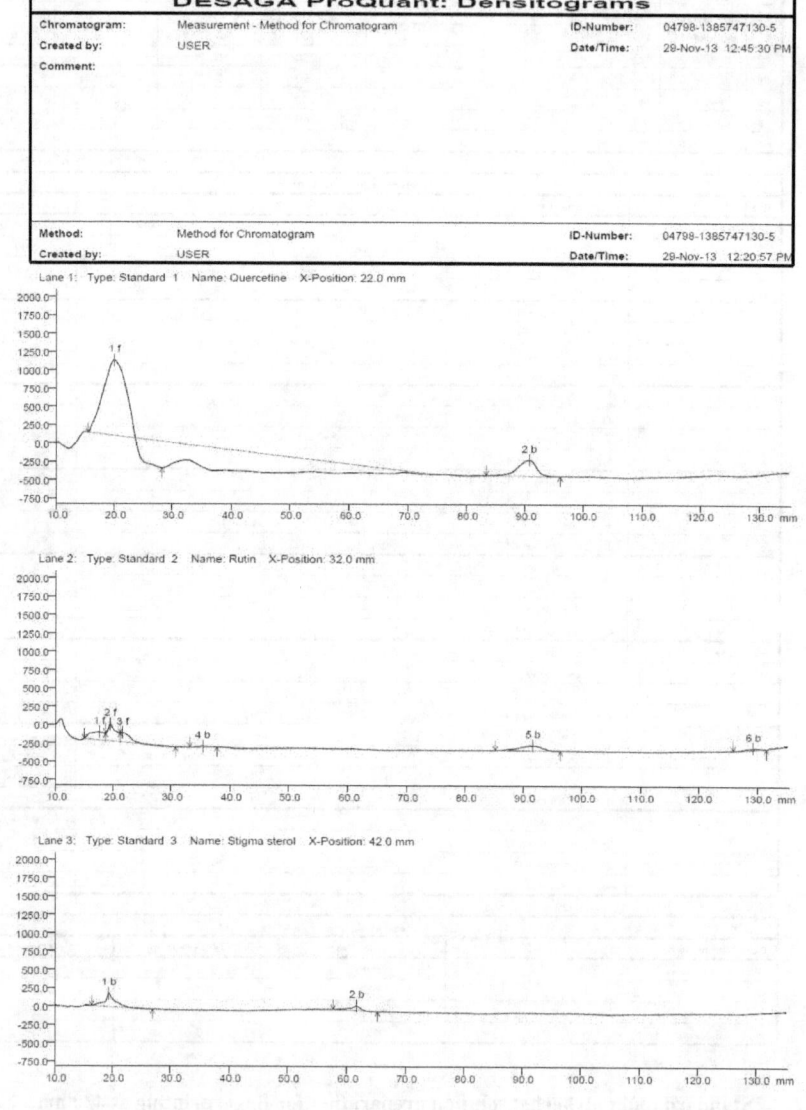

Figure 5.50: Chromatogram of Quercetin, Rutin and Stigma sterol at 420 nm

Chapter 5 Results and Observations

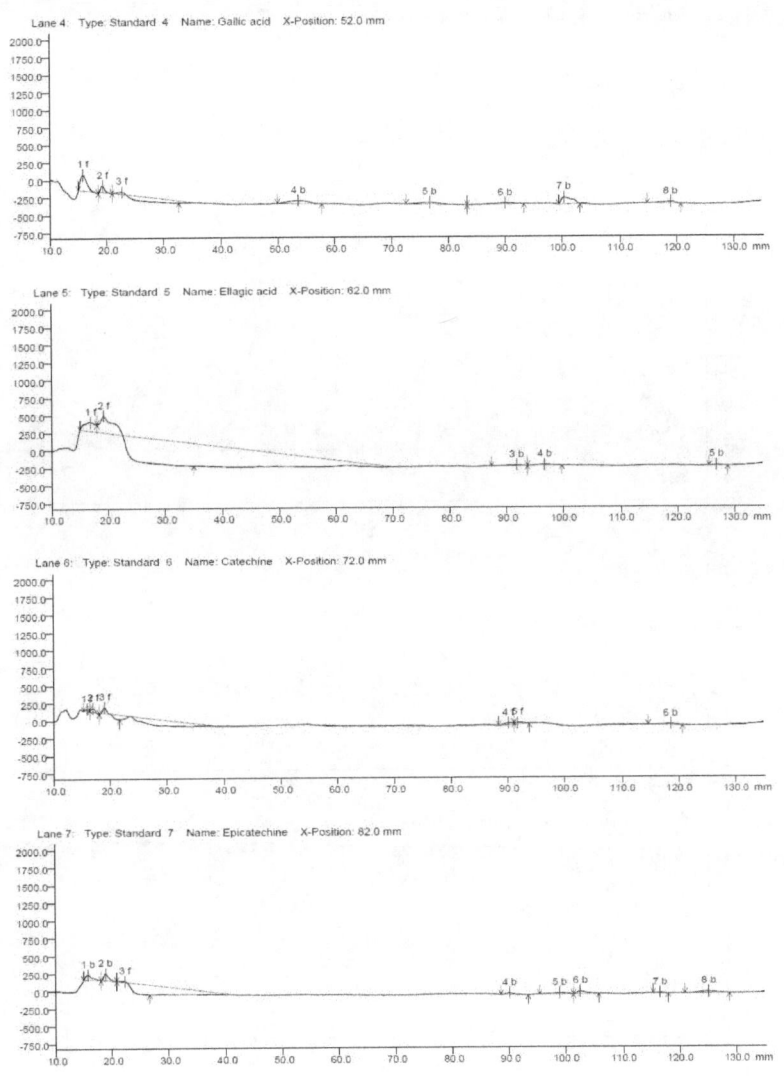

Figure 5.51: Chromatogram of Gallic acid, Ellagic acid, Catechin and Epicatechin at 420 nm

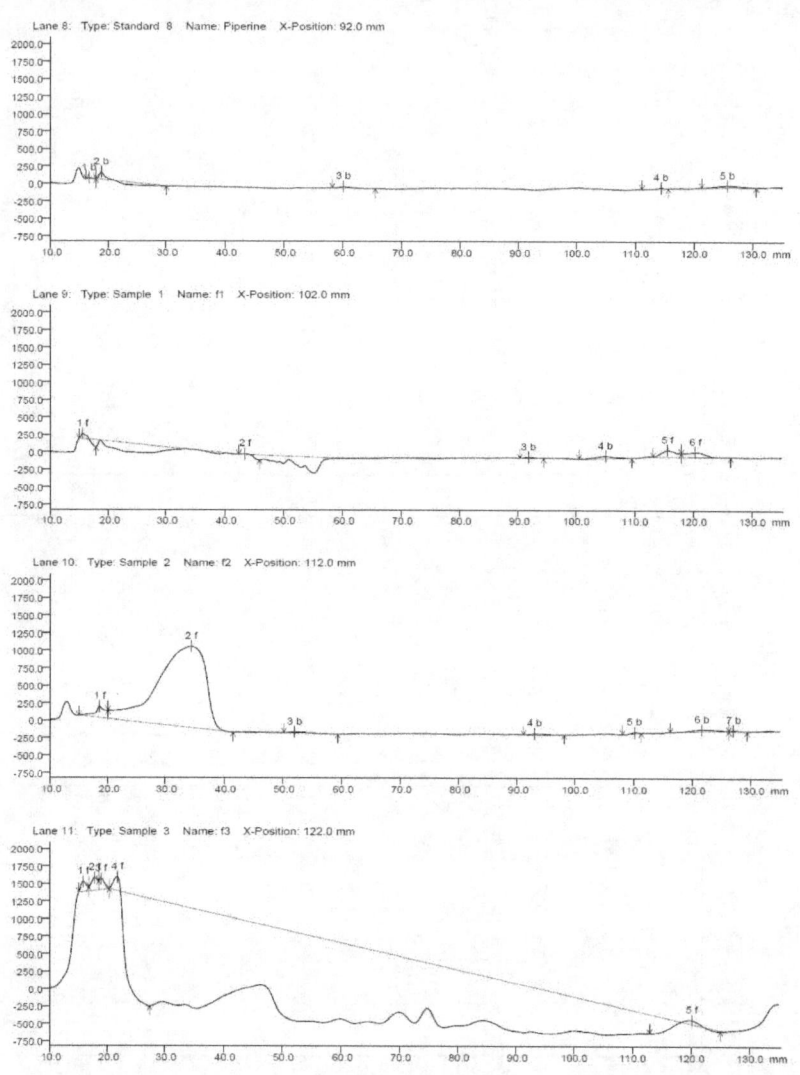

Figure 5.52: Chromatogram of Piperine, Polyherbal FA (f1), FB (f2) and FC (f3) at 420 nm

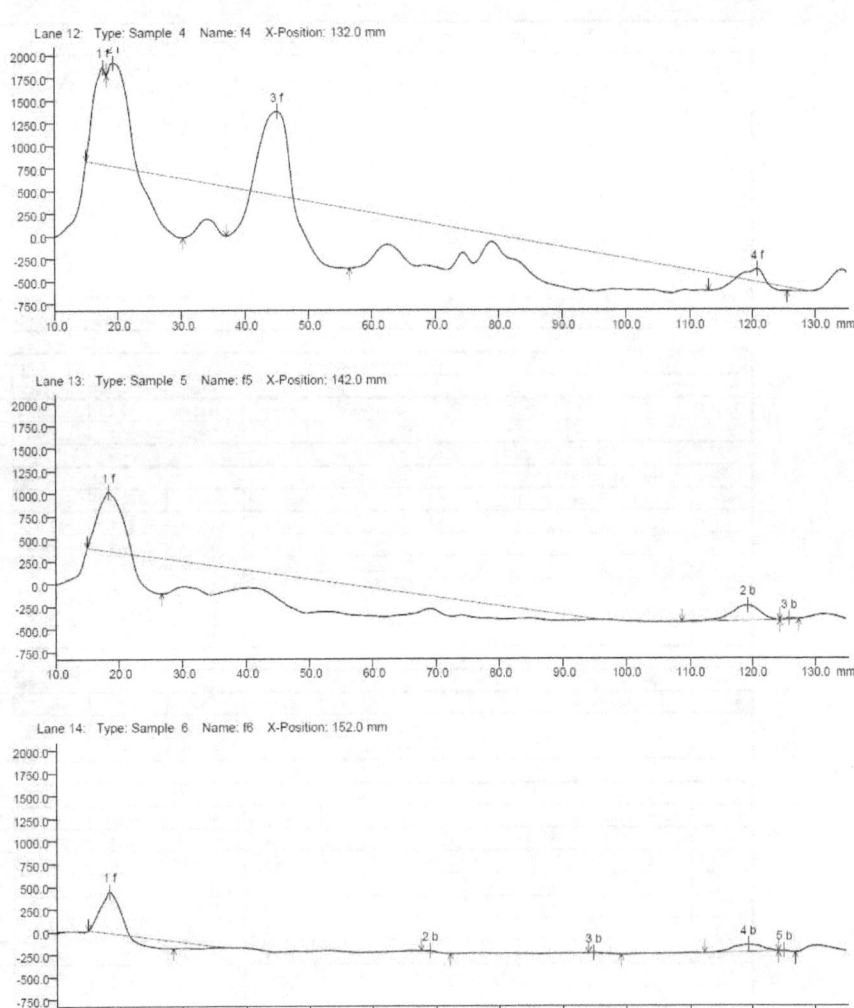

Figure 5.53: Chromatogram of Polyherbal FD (f4), FE (f5) and FF (f6) at 420 nm

DESAGA ProQuant: Peak list

Chromatogram:	Measurement - Method for Chromatogram	ID-Number:	04798-1385747130-5
Created by:	USER	Date/Time:	29-Nov-13 12:45:30 PM
Comment:			

Method:	Method for Chromatogram	ID-Number:	04798-1385747130-5
Created by:	USER	Date/Time:	29-Nov-13 12:20:57 PM

Lane: 1   Type: Standard 1   Name: Quercetin   X-Position: 22.0 mm

Peak	Component name		y-Pos [mm]	Area	Area[%]	Height	Type	Rf
1	:	Quercetin	20.0	4577.05	85.2	1025.07	f	0.04
2	:		90.7	797.84	14.8	216.34	b	0.63

Lane: 2   Type: Standard 2   Name: Rutin   X-Position: 32.0 mm

Peak	Component name		y-Pos [mm]	Area	Area[%]	Height	Type	Rf
1	:		17.6	297.11	23.2	107.37	f	0.02
2	:		19.5	369.30	28.9	229.35	f	0.04
3	:	Rutin	21.6	224.12	17.5	126.59	f	0.06
4	:		35.4	19.29	1.5	10.73	b	0.17
5	:		91.6	316.13	24.7	70.27	b	0.64
6	:		129.2	53.59	4.2	19.40	b	0.95

Lane: 3   Type: Standard 3   Name: Stigma sterol   X-Position: 42.0 mm

Peak	Component name		y-Pos [mm]	Area	Area[%]	Height	Type	Rf
1	:		19.4	357.95	74.1	178.56	b	0.04
2	:	Stigma sterol	61.7	124.86	25.9	64.13	b	0.39

Lane: 4   Type: Standard 4   Name: Gallic acid   X-Position: 52.0 mm

Peak	Component name		y-Pos [mm]	Area	Area[%]	Height	Type	Rf
1	:		15.8	287.81	27.7	219.97	f	0.01
2	:		19.3	70.18	6.8	92.69	f	0.04
3	:		22.7	43.29	4.2	30.20	f	0.06
4	:		53.6	174.53	16.8	41.13	b	0.32
5	:		76.7	113.01	10.9	29.08	b	0.51
6	:		90.0	61.10	5.9	15.34	b	0.62
7	:	Gallic acid	100.3	217.90	21.0	102.99	b	0.71
8	:		118.9	69.94	6.7	28.09	b	0.87

Lane: 5   Type: Standard 5   Name: Ellagic acid   X-Position: 62.0 mm

Peak	Component name		y-Pos [mm]	Area	Area[%]	Height	Type	Rf
1	:		16.9	294.65	28.0	126.97	f	0.02
2	:		19.2	678.26	64.5	242.51	f	0.04
3	:		91.8	27.04	2.6	10.05	b	0.64
4	:	Ellagic acid	96.7	39.85	3.8	11.99	b	0.68
5	:		126.7	11.60	1.1	10.62	b	0.93

Chapter 5 — Results and Observations

Lane: 6	Type: Standard 6		Name: Catechine			X-Position: 72.0 mm		
Peak	Component name			y-Pos [mm]	Area	Area[%]	Height	Type	Rf
1	:			15.9	20.92	8.8	27.30	f	0.01
2	:			17.0	40.08	16.8	51.02	f	0.02
3	:			19.1	59.30	24.9	80.96	f	0.03
4	:		Catechine	90.1	46.77	19.6	26.66	f	0.63
5	:			91.7	39.48	16.6	22.01	f	0.64
6	:			118.5	31.75	13.3	14.29	b	0.86

Lane: 7	Type: Standard 7		Name: Epicatechine			X-Position: 82.0 mm		
Peak	Component name			y-Pos [mm]	Area	Area[%]	Height	Type	Rf
1	:			15.8	101.70	21.1	75.68	b	0.01
2	:			18.9	99.66	20.7	102.32	b	0.03
3	:			22.3	11.77	2.4	11.14	f	0.06
4	:			90.1	39.71	8.2	22.13	b	0.63
5	:			98.9	54.67	11.4	16.51	b	0.70
6	:			102.5	71.92	14.9	39.92	b	0.73
7	:			116.5	12.22	2.5	10.58	b	0.85
8	:		Epicatechine	125.0	89.90	18.7	24.88	b	0.92

Lane: 8	Type: Standard 8		Name: Piperine			X-Position: 92.0 mm		
Peak	Component name			y-Pos [mm]	Area	Area[%]	Height	Type	Rf
1	:			16.7	11.13	3.8	14.24	b	0.01
2	:			18.8	112.37	37.9	105.09	b	0.03
3	:			60.1	45.99	15.5	18.57	b	0.38
4	:			114.3	14.59	4.9	10.83	b	0.83
5	:		Piperine	125.6	112.55	37.9	25.57	b	0.92

Lane: 9	Type: Sample 1		Name: f1			X-Position: 102.0 mm		
Peak	Component name			y-Pos [mm]	Area	Area[%]	Height	Type	Rf
1	:			15.6	73.26	9.5	68.15	f	0.01
2	:			43.5	12.52	1.6	10.36	f	0.24
3	:		Catechine	91.8	22.75	2.9	13.14	b	0.64
4	:		Gallic acid	105.0	117.17	15.1	33.20	b	0.73
5	:			115.5	281.42	36.3	94.84	f	0.84
6	:			120.3	267.77	34.6	67.23	f	0.88

Lane: 10	Type: Sample 2		Name: f2			X-Position: 112.0 mm		
Peak	Component name			y-Pos [mm]	Area	Area[%]	Height	Type	Rf
1	:		Quercetin	18.6	345.89	3.0	163.30	f	0.03
2	:			34.4	10927.96	94.8	1162.85	f	0.16
3	:			52.0	48.92	0.4	11.46	b	0.31
4	:		Catechine	93.0	49.13	0.4	14.22	b	0.65
5	:			110.1	17.34	0.2	13.98	b	0.79
6	:			121.6	130.59	1.1	28.42	b	0.89
7	:		Epicatechine ,Piperine	127.0	12.27	0.1	11.71	b	0.93

Lane: 11	Type: Sample 3		Name: f3			X-Position: 122.0 mm		
Peak	Component name			y-Pos [mm]	Area	Area[%]	Height	Type	Rf
1	:			15.8	169.40	18.5	146.31	f	0.01
2	:			17.8	224.96	24.5	183.84	f	0.02
3	:		Quercetin	18.9	159.21	17.4	152.95	f	0.03
4	:		Rutin	21.7	222.58	24.3	197.66	f	0.06

| 5 | : | | 120.1 | 141.19 | 15.4 | 57.39 | f | 0.88 |

Lane: 12　　Type: Sample 4　　Name: f4　　　　　　　　　　　　　　X-Position: 132.0 mm

Peak	Component name		y-Pos [mm]	Area	Area[%]	Height	Type	Rf
1	:		17.7	2337.83	21.7	1069.65	f	0.02
2	:	Quercetin	19.4	3878.55	35.9	1140.11	f	0.04
3	:		45.1	4165.12	38.6	926.72	f	0.25
4	:		120.8	410.62	3.8	141.56	f	0.88

Lane: 13　　Type: Sample 5　　Name: f5　　　　　　　　　　　　　　X-Position: 142.0 mm

Peak	Component name		y-Pos [mm]	Area	Area[%]	Height	Type	Rf
1	:	Quercetin	18.4	2792.37	75.0	651.12	f	0.03
2	:		119.2	911.07	24.5	169.47	b	0.87
3	:	Epicatechine, Piperine	125.8	17.65	0.5	14.05	b	0.92

Lane: 14　　Type: Sample 6　　Name: f6　　　　　　　　　　　　　　X-Position: 152.0 mm

Peak	Component name		y-Pos [mm]	Area	Area[%]	Height	Type	Rf
1	:	Quercetin	18.4	1585.25	76.7	457.24	f	0.03
2	:		69.0	18.09	0.9	11.27	b	0.45
3	:	Ellagic acid	94.7	24.78	1.2	10.09	b	0.66
4	:		119.3	427.43	20.7	78.66	b	0.87
5	:	Epicatechine, Piperine	125.0	10.52	0.5	10.16	b	0.92

Figure 5.54: Peak list of Standards and Polyherbal Formulations at 420 nm

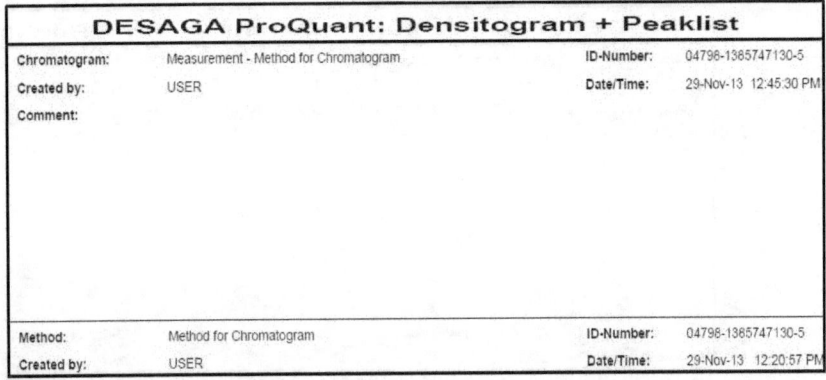
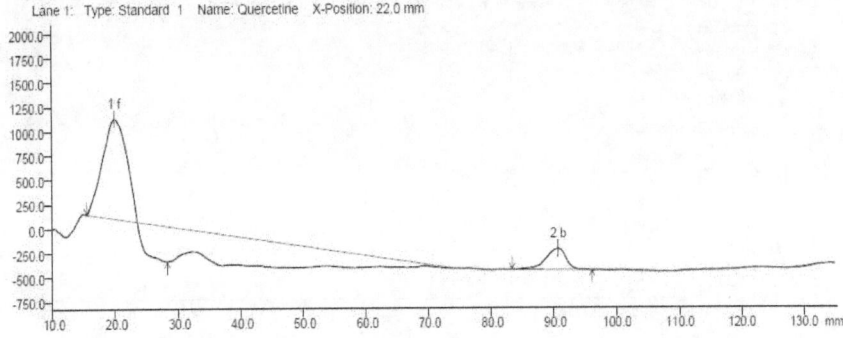

Figure 5.55: Chromatogram of Quercetin at 420 nm

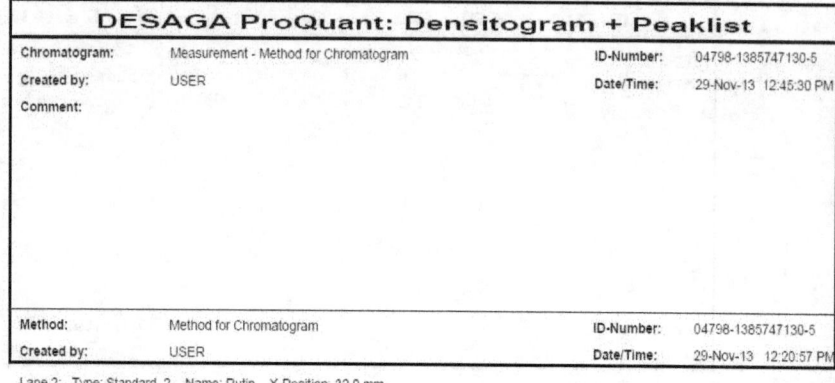

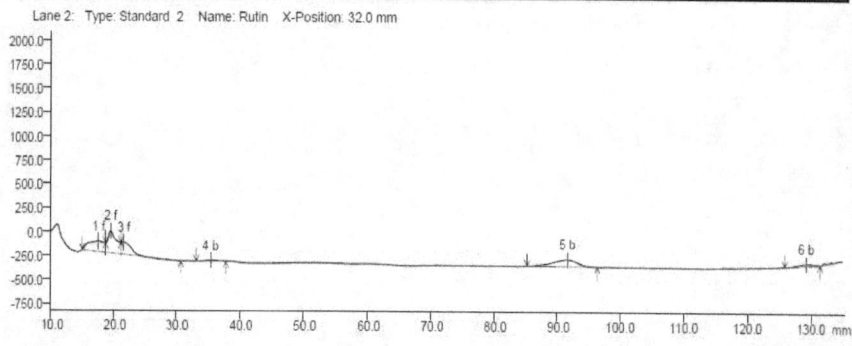

Peak	Component name	y-Pos [mm]	Area	Area[%]	Height	Type	Rf
1	:	17.6	297.11	23.2	107.37	f	0.02
2	:	19.5	369.30	28.9	229.35	f	0.04
3	:	21.6	224.12	17.5	126.59	f	0.06
4	:	35.4	19.29	1.5	10.73	b	0.17
5	:	91.6	316.13	24.7	70.27	b	0.64
6	:	129.2	53.59	4.2	19.40	b	0.95

Figure 5.56: Chromatogram of Rutin at 420 nm

Chapter 5 — Results and Observations

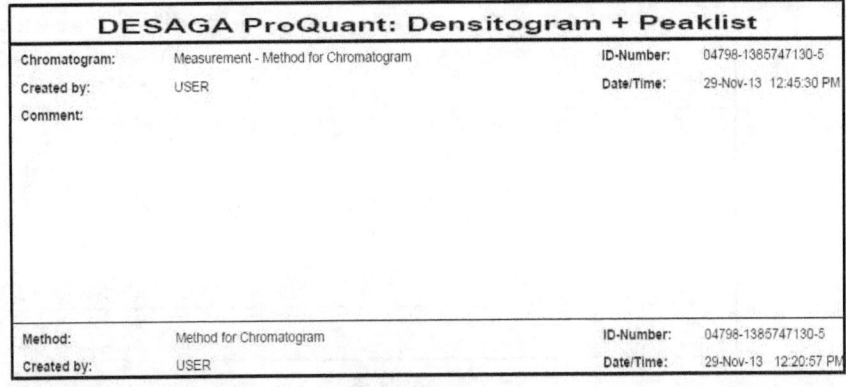

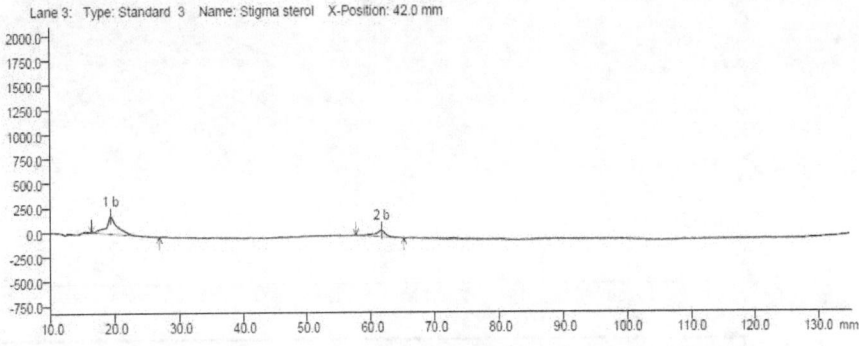

Lane: 3	Type: Standard 3		Name: Stigma sterol				X-Position: 42.0 mm	
Peak	Component name		y-Pos [mm]	Area	Area[%]	Height	Type	Rf
1	:		19.4	357.95	74.1	178.56	b	0.04
2	:		61.7	124.86	25.9	64.13	b	0.39

Figure 5.57: Chromatogram of Stigma sterol at 420 nm

Chapter 5 — Results and Observations

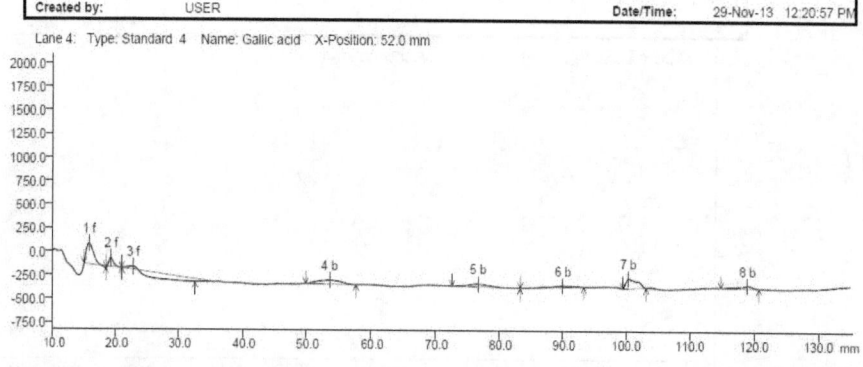

Figure 5.58: Chromatogram of Gallic acid at 420 nm

Chapter 5   Results and Observations

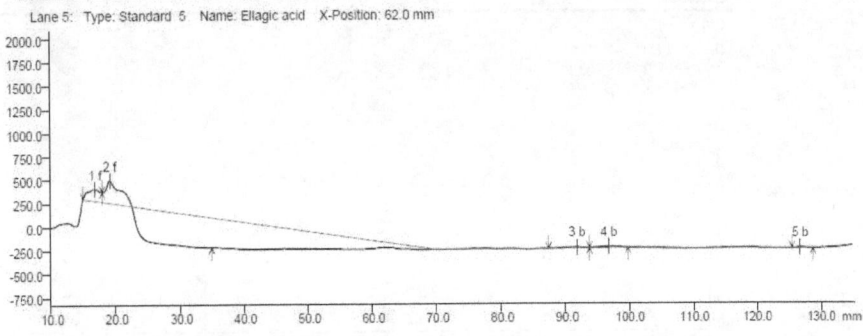

Figure 5.59: Chromatogram of Ellagic acid at 420 nm

DESAGA ProQuant: Densitogram + Peaklist

Chromatogram:	Measurement - Method for Chromatogram	ID-Number:	04798-1385747130-5
Created by:	USER	Date/Time:	29-Nov-13 12:45:30 PM
Comment:			

Method:	Method for Chromatogram	ID-Number:	04798-1385747130-5
Created by:	USER	Date/Time:	29-Nov-13 12:20:57 PM

Lane 6: Type: Standard 6   Name: Catechine   X-Position: 72.0 mm

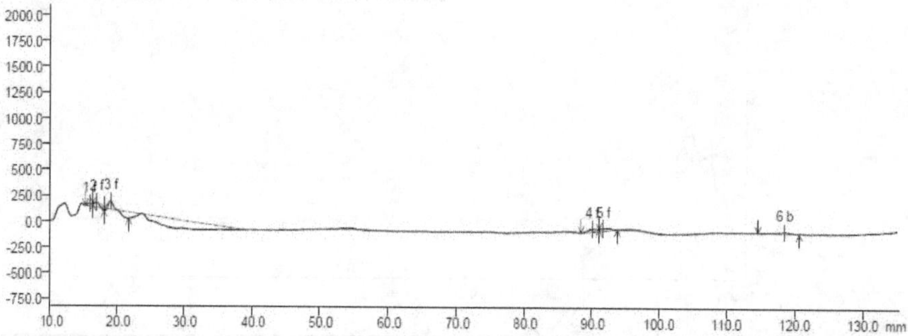

Lane: 6   Type: Standard 6   Name: Catechine   X-Position: 72.0 mm

Peak	Component name	y-Pos [mm]	Area	Area[%]	Height	Type	Rf
1	:	15.9	20.92	8.8	27.30	f	0.01
2	:	17.0	40.08	16.8	51.02	f	0.02
3	:	19.1	59.30	24.9	80.96	f	0.03
4	:	90.1	46.77	19.6	26.66	f	0.63
5	:	91.7	39.48	16.6	22.01	f	0.64
6	:	118.5	31.75	13.3	14.29	b	0.86

Figure 5.60: Chromatogram of Catechin acid at 420 nm

Chapter 5   Results and Observations

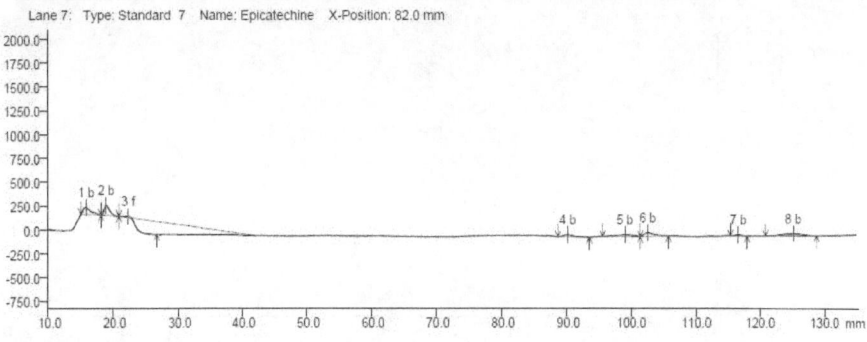

Figure 5.61: Chromatogram of Epicatechin acid at 420 nm

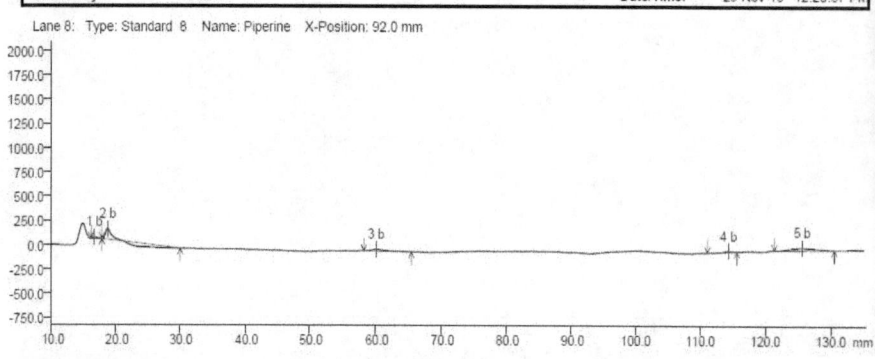

Figure 5.62: Chromatogram of Piperine acid at 420 nm

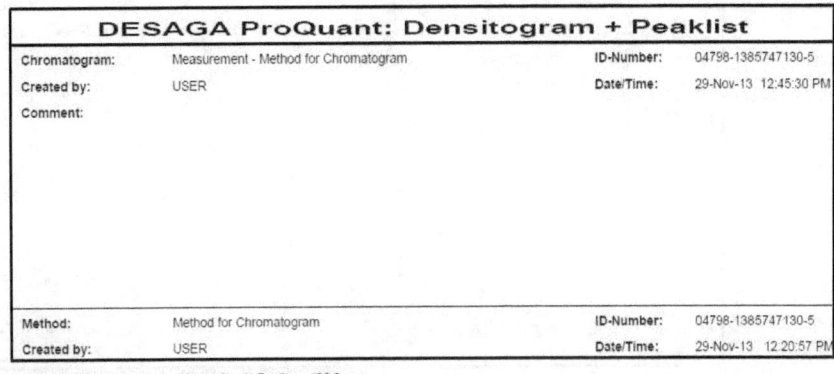

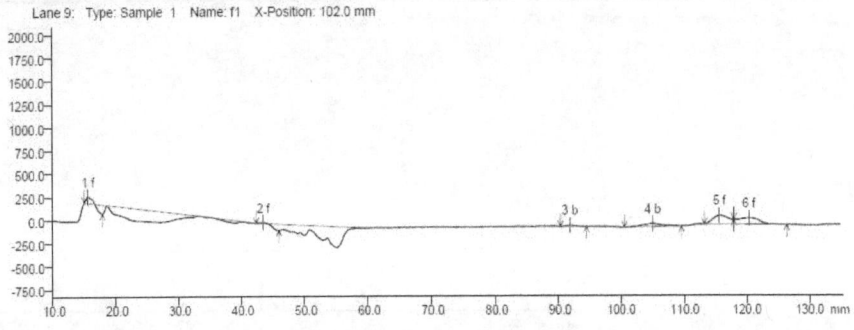

Figure 5.63: Chromatogram of Polyherbal formulation FA (f1) at 420 nm

Chapter 5 — Results and Observations

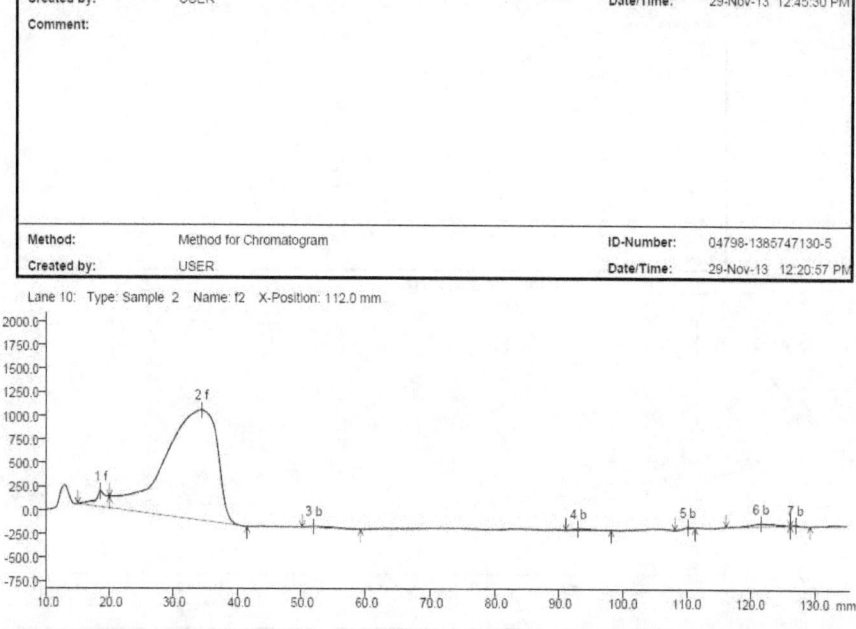

Figure 5.64: Chromatogram of Polyherbal formulation FB (f2) at 420 nm

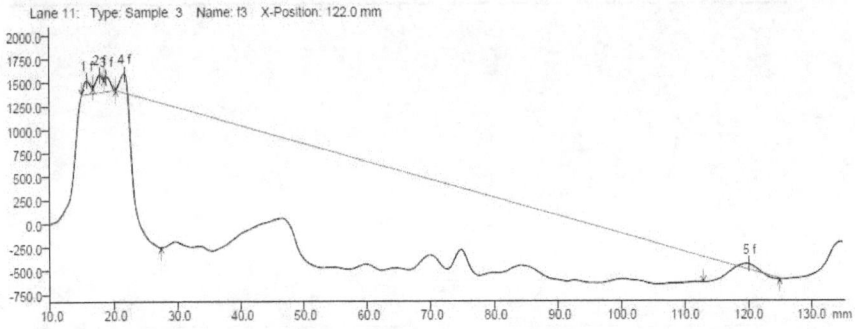

Figure 5.65: Chromatogram of Polyherbal formulation FC (f3) at 420 nm

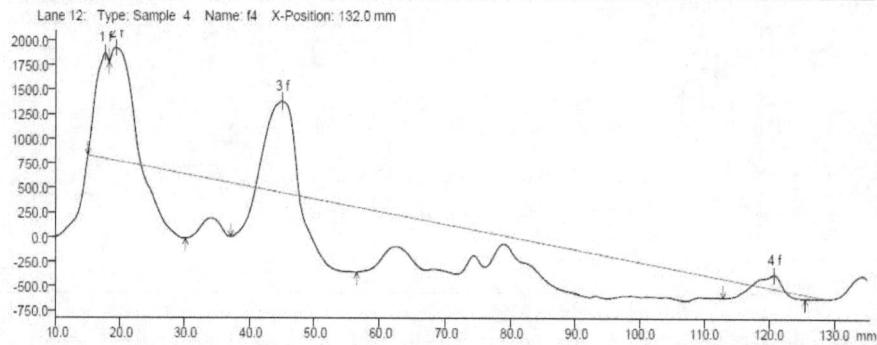

Figure 5.66: Chromatogram of Polyherbal formulation FD (f4) at 420 nm

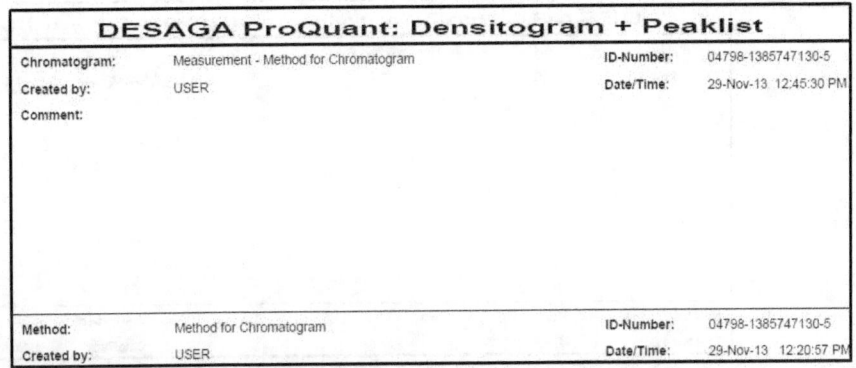
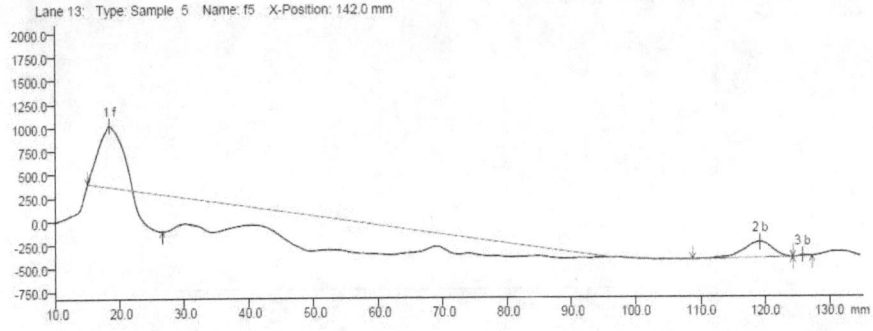

Figure 5.67: Chromatogram of Polyherbal formulation FE (f5) at 420 nm

DESAGA ProQuant: Densitogram + Peaklist

Chromatogram:	Measurement - Method for Chromatogram	ID-Number:	04798-1385747130-5
Created by:	USER	Date/Time:	29-Nov-13 12:45:30 PM
Comment:			

Method:	Method for Chromatogram	ID-Number:	04798-1385747130-5
Created by:	USER	Date/Time:	29-Nov-13 12:20:57 PM

Lane 14: Type: Sample 6 Name: f6 X-Position: 152.0 mm

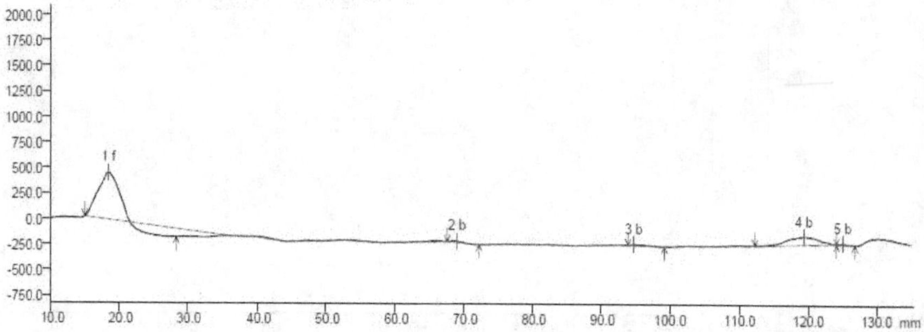

Lane: 14 Type: Sample 6 Name: f6 X-Position: 152.0 mm

Peak	Component name	y-Pos [mm]	Area	Area[%]	Height	Type	Rf
1	:	18.4	1585.25	76.7	457.24	f	0.03
2	:	69.0	18.09	0.9	11.27	b	0.45
3	:	94.7	24.78	1.2	10.09	b	0.66
4	:	119.3	427.43	20.7	78.66	b	0.87
5	:	125.0	10.52	0.5	10.16	b	0.92

Figure 5.68: Chromatogram of Polyherbal formulation FF (f6) at 420 nm

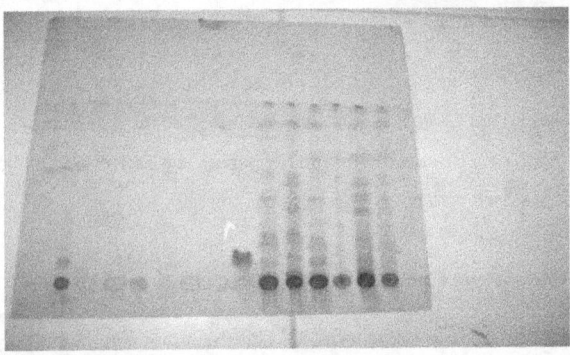

Figure 5.69: TLC of Polyherbal Formulations with Standards at 420 nm

5.8.2 Safety assessment

Results of toxicity study are already discussed and results showed that higher dose of 2000 mg/kg b.wt did not cause any mortality and therefore the formulations were found to be safe on acute exposure. Results of other safety parameters i.e Heavy metal content determination and microbial load are shown in tables 5.27 and 5.28

5.8.2.1 Heavy Metal Content Determination

The content of Arsenic, Mercury, Lead and Cadmium was found to be within permissible limits as laid down by guidelines for quality standardized herbal formulations of WHO as shown in table 5.27. Mercury and Cadmium was not detected in all the Polyherbals and Arsenic was not detected in formulation A, C and F.

Table 5.27: Results of Heavy metal content determination in Polyherbal formulations by Atomic absorption Spectroscopy.

Polyherbal	Lead (µg/ml)	Cadmium (µg/ml)	Mercury (µg/ml)	Arsenic (µg/ml)
A	1.7	Not Detected	Not Detected	Not Detected
B	3.6	Not Detected	Not Detected	0.2
C	4.0	Not Detected	Not Detected	Not Detected
D	2.8	Not Detected	Not Detected	0.7
E	1.2	Not Detected	Not Detected	0.3
F	1.8	Not Detected	Not Detected	Not Detected

5.8.2.2 Microbial load

Results of microbial load (fungi and bacteria) in all the Polyherbals was found to be within limits as prescribed in WHO guidelines as shown in table 5.28.

Table 5.28: Results of Microbial Load in Polyherbal Formulation (FA-FF)

Polyherbals	Method	Bacteria count	Fungi count
A		Less than 10^1 CFU/ml	2×10^1 CFU/ml
B		Less than 10^1 CFU/ml	2×10^1 CFU/ml
C	A.P.I 2.4.1	Less than 10^1 CFU/ml	2×10^1 CFU/ml
D		Less than 10^1 CFU/ml	2×10^1 CFU/ml
E		Less than 10^1 CFU/ml	2×10^1 CFU/ml
F		Less than 10^1 CFU/ml	2×10^1 CFU/ml

CHAPTER-6

Discussion

Chapter 6 — Discussion

Since the prehistoric time herbal medicines have existed worldwide with the long healing history. Since 19th century with the increase in availability of chemical analytical techniques, developments of herbal remedies are progressing for various therapeutic purposes and diseases. Although synthetic routes of medicines have strong pharmacological actions but due to numerous side-effects and lack of medicines to chronic ailments, masses are shifting back to herbals drugs and led to re-emergence of herbal medicines.

Most of diseases like diabetes, heart disease, cancer and psychiatric disorders are multifactorial and need more therapeutic interventions at more than one level. Diabetes is one such disease that has become serious problem of modern society due to its health complications, undesirable side effects arises from the use of synthetic drugs in the disease. Plants with complex phytochemical mixtures have advantage in treating such diseases being devoid of toxic side-effects. Although most of the individual plant constituents have been established and served for the treatment of disease but they are usually present in minute amount and lacking to achieve the desirable side effects. Hence scientifically the combination methodology of different plants with varying potency was proved successful and also helps in maintaining the loophole of individual plant drug treatment as these methodologies produce greater and effective results as compare to individual use of plants. Hence this combination methodology called as herb-herb interaction (synergism). Herb-Herb interaction in polyherbal are depends on two mechanism pharmacokinetic synergism (ability to facilitate ADME of other herb) and pharmacodynamics synergism. It is believed that polyherbal formulations act on the multiple targets at the same time. Hence multiple component formulation (polyherbal formulations) gives better therapeutic effects than single plant drug.

All the six formulations (FA, FB, FC, FD, FE and FF) have been developed with combinations of (only emerging antidiabetic plants, only traditional antidiabetic plants and mixture of traditional and emerging plants. Antidiabetic activity was investigated in albino wistar rats with glibenclamide as standard, STZ was used to induce diabetes in rats. All the Polyherbals showed significant decrease in Blood glucose level with improvement in slight loss of body weight. Albino wistar rats were divided in XV groups with n=5 and the diabetic rats received all the formulations (FA, FB, FC, FD, FE, and FF), vehicle and standard drug. Although all the formulations showed good antidiabetic activity but FD (400 mg/kg) against diabetes very efficient in all six Polyherbals. Polyherbal FD consists of amalgamation of only emerging antidiabetic plants in fixed doses of each extracts. It showed 65.8% decrease in average blood glucose level which was very closer to standard drug glibenclamide. i.e. 66.2%. Reason for this superior activity of FD may be its potential active constituents which could possess better antidiabetic activity and the second main reason may its synergism (herb-herb interactions) which may be more compatible when formulated together in polyherbal and thus produce more effective results.

As mentioned in results all the formulations gives dose dependent antidiabetic effect but in polyherbal formulation FF lower dose (200 mg) was more effective in reducing blood glucose level as compared to higher dose (400 mg). Polyherbal A, B, C which is a combination of both the traditional and emerging medicinal plants, in these combinations B was proved to be fruitful and comparable to standard against glibenclamide.

Rest of 3 combinations contains equal quantity of plant extract. In these combination polyherbal D was more effective as an antidiabetic formulation medicine. With equal dose of plant extract in polyherbal E (combination of traditional plant extract) also showed good antidiabetic activity with dose of 400 mg (i.e. 62.4 %) decrease in blood glucose level.

On the basis of best synergistic effect FD>FB>FE>FC>FF>FA

All the lipid content except HDL (which was increased) was found to be increased in STZ diabetic rats. HDL- Cholesterol was found to be more increased in FD and FF combination as compared to others. All combinations improve the conditions of hypercholesterolemia. FD combination showed a greater increase in HDL % level to 57.12 % than those of std. glibenclamide. In polyherbal E and F no satisfactory reduction was observed for lipid profile except HDL and LDL level which was observed to be somewhat satisfactory.

It has been observed through literatures that plants constituents like glycosides, alkaloids, flavonoids all these constituents have proved to be strong antidiabetic agent through different mechanism.

1) By increasing the uptake of glucose through specific receptors (*Annona squamosa*)
2) By inhibiting alpha amylase enzyme (*Morus alba*).

3) Inhibiting the glucose-6-phosphatase, gluconeogenic enzyme therapy increasing the insulin secretion from β-cell of pancreas (*Coccinia indica*).
4) Increasing the insulin secretion from the β cell pf pancreas.
5) Re-generation of β cell of pancreas (*Gymnea sylvestre*)
6) As bioavailability enhancer (*Piper longum*)

HPTLC Fingerprinting confirmed the presence of compounds i.e Gallic acid, Quercetin, Catechin, Piperine, Rutin, Stigma sterol. Literatures have already been described the antidiabetic effect of these compounds and even in some countries these compounds have been confirmed as standard antidiabetic compounds. Since all the polyherbal contain many active phytoconstituents, it is difficult to find out the exact single mechanism for antidiabetic effect as phytoconstituents Rutin inhibit the alpha amylase enzyme, Catechin modulates the secretion of insulin, Quercetin increases the glucose uptake by tissues and Piperine is well known for its bioavailability enhancing availability in many polyherbal formulations. So multicomponent formulations targeted the multiple sites for its antidiabetic action at a single time and hence succeeded in producing the synergistic antidiabetic effect and reduce the side effects.

CHAPTER-7

Conclusion and direction for future use

Chapter 7 — Conclusion and Direction for Future Use

Since Ancient times medicinal plants as single drug and in combination with other herbal drugs are using in the treatment of various chronic and non-chronic disorders. Ayurveda is one of the most traditional systems of medicine which describes the methodology to use the medicinal plants as healing power in treating the disease. Polyherbalism is also the best concept of Ayurveda, which consists of magical power of healing the disease. Ayurveda is one of the reliable and trustworthy medicine systems. In developing countries mostly 75-95% of populations rely on herbal drugs. Deep research and investigation still needed on this magical system of medicines. Research Studies pertaining to safety, toxicological studies, Standardization, clinical trial studies are still required to grow Ayurveda and increasing its wide acceptability. Numbers of commercialized standardized herbal drugs arequiet less in market since we are lacking in developing the regulatory standards implemented protocols.

Diabetes mellitus has appearing as dreadful disorder for society. It directly impacts our metabolic system by making it sluggish in catabolic activities. It is mainly characterized by hyperglycemia resulted from decrease insulin secretion. This dreadful disease can lead to many more complications like blindness, kidney failure and organ dysfunction.

Several synthetic drugs are available in market but with long use of these drugs could lead to serious side effect including the kidney failure there is greater risk of using these synthetic drugs for long term.

Study of ancient Ayurvedic books like *Charak Samhita* and *Sushastra Samhita* revealed that drugs used in Ayurvedic formulations worked synergistically on root cause of disease. Therefore a quality control drug will be effective in management of diabetes.

Commercially available antidiabetic herbal formulations used well known medicinal plants like *Momordica charantia, Syzium cumini, Coccinia indica, Pterocarpus marsupium, Piper longum, Gymnea sylvestre* however there are number of new plants which have been proved be potential antidiabetic drugs and their mode of action have been established by large number of scientist. Some of such emerging antidiabetic plants are *Annona squamosa, Morusalba, Psidium guajava, Nelumbo nucifera*.

Chapter 7 — Conclusion and Direction for Future Use

In view of above 5 drugs from traditionally used and 5 drugs from list of emerging antidiabetic plants drugs, based on their reported mode of action six different formulations were made by using extracts of (5 plants) of both traditional and emerging antidiabetic drugs.

All the six formulations were subjected to acute toxicity study and fount to be safe up to dose of 2000 mg/kg b.wt. After this glucose tolerance test (OGTT) was performed in animal model for preliminary assessment of antidiabetic activity.

The antidiabetic activity was studied in albino wistar rats as per standard protocol. The diabetes was induced by use of Streptozotocin (STZ). For the study of antidiabetic activity all the six formulations were given in 2 doses of 200 mg/kg b.wt and 400 mg/kg b.wt. for 15 days.

The blood samples of each rat were analyzed for various biochemical parameters. The results showed that formulations FD containing extracts of (*Annona squamosa*, *Morus alba*, *Nelumbo nucifera*, *Piper longum* and *Psidium guajava*) showed significant antidiabetic activity which was close to standard drug. Along with remarkable reduction in Total Cholesterol (TC) level and increased in High Density Lipoprotein (HDL) Streptozotocin induced diabetes rats. The formulation has emerged as potential combination which can challenge the synthetic drug.

Second combination FB (containing combination of traditionally used as well as emerging antidiabetic drugs) also proved to have significant antidiabetic activity when compared with standard drug the glibenclamide. Here we can summarize the decreasing order of significant effect of antidiabetic activity polyherbal formulations FD>FB>FE>FC>FF>FA.

Studies for Quality control and safety of product was also performed, some of the constituents of the plants are also identified in formulations like Gallic acid, Piperine, Rutin and Ellagic acid. Gallic acid. Gallic acid stimulates glucose uptake by inducing GLUT4 translocation and facilities the glucose absorption. Piperine was known for its bio enhancing property. Previous study showed that rutin decreased glycemia, serum insulin concentration and liver glycogen content and hexokinase activities. Rutin was also effective in improving muscle insulin sensitivity by increasing the expression of the receptor PPAR-γ Quercetin has been known to increase the hepatic glucokinase activity and also help in regeneration of pancreatic islet cells. Therefore for quality control HPTLC study was performed using above compounds as marker.

For safety studies of formulations microbial load (Total Bacterial count and Total Fungal count) and heavy metal content were determined and the formulation was found to be safe.

The study revealed that out of 6 formulations FD containing only emerging antidiabetic plants like *Annona squamosa, Morus alba, Nelumbo nucifera, Psidium guajava* was capable of reducing sugar level almost equal to modern drug glibenclamide. Formulation FB containing combination of traditionally used as well as emerging antidiabetic drugs has also shown significant antidiabetic activity which was comparable to modern drug.

Future Perspectives: The above formulations FD and FB may be taken up for clinical trial as per standard protocol and guidelines. After clinical study drug can be taken up pharmaceutical companies for commercial exploitation. All the plant materials of FD and FB groups are very common in natural occurrence and their availability for commercial exploitation will not be any problem.

www.ingramcontent.com/pod-product-compliance
Lightning Source LLC
Chambersburg PA
CBHW050206230526
45470CB00001B/265